Obesity and Diabetes in Sports Medicine

Guest Editors

SUSAN E. KIRK, MD
DILAAWAR J. MISTRY, MD, MS, ATC

CLINICS IN SPORTS MEDICINE

www.sportsmed.theclinics.com

Consulting Editor
MARK D. MILLER, MD

July 2009 • Volume 28 • Number 3

SAUNDERS an imprint of ELSEVIER, Inc.

W.B. SAUNDERS COMPANY
A Division of Elsevier Inc.

1600 John F. Kennedy Blvd. • Suite 1800 • Philadelphia, Pennsylvania 19103

http://www.theclinics.com

CLINICS IN SPORTS MEDICINE Volume 28, Number 3
July 2009 ISSN 0278-5919, ISBN-13: 978-1-4377-1275-9, ISBN-10: 1-4377-1275-4

Editor: Ruth Malwitz
Developmental Editor: Theresa Collier

Clinics in Sports Medicine (ISSN 0278-5919) is published quarterly by Elsevier Inc., 360 Park Avenue South, New York, NY 10010-1710. Months of publication are January, April, July, and October. Business and Editorial Offices: 1600 John F. Kennedy Blvd., Suite 1800, Philadelphia, PA 19103-2899. Customer Service Offices: 6277 Sea Harbor Drive, Orlando, FL 32887-4800. Periodicals postage paid at New York, NY, and additional mailing offices. Subscription prices are $253.00 per year (US individuals), $393.00 per year (US institutions), $127.00 per year (US students), $286.00 per year (Canadian individuals), $475.00 per year (Canadian institutions), $177.00 (Canadian students), $347.00 per year (foreign individuals), $475.00 per year (foreign institutions), and $177.00 per year (foreign students). Foreign air speed delivery is included in all *Clinics* subscription prices. All prices are subject to change without notice. **POSTMASTER:** Send address changes to *Clinics in Sports Medicine*, Elsevier Periodicals Customer Service, 11830 Westline Industrial Drive, St. Louis, MO 63146. Customer Service (orders, claims, online, change of address): Elsevier Periodicals Customer Service, 11830 Westline Industrial Drive, St. Louis, MO 63146. Tel: 1-800-654-2452 (U.S. and Canada); 314-453-7041 (outside U.S. and Canada). Fax: 314-453-5170. E-mail: journalscustomerservice-usa@elsevier.com (for print support); journalsonlinesupport-usa@elsevier.com (for online support).

Reprints. For copies of 100 or more of articles in this publication, please contact the Commercial Reprints Department, Elsevier Inc., 360 Park Avenue South, New York, NY 10010-1710. Tel.: 212-633-3812; Fax: 212-462-1935; E-mail: reprints@elsevier.com.

Clinics in Sports Medicine is covered in *MEDLINE/PubMed (Index Medicus) Current Contents/Clinical Medicine, Excerpta Medica,* and *ISI/Biomed.*

Printed and bound by CPI Group (UK) Ltd, Croydon, CR0 4YY

Transferred to Digital Print 2012

Contributors

CONSULTING EDITOR

MARK D. MILLER, MD
S. Ward Casscells Professor of Orthopaedic Surgery; Head, Division of Sports Medicine, University of Virginia; Team Physician, James Madison University, Charlottesville, Virginia

GUEST EDITORS

SUSAN E. KIRK, MD
Associate Professor of Internal Medicine and Obstetrics and Gynecology, Division of Endocrinology and Metabolism; Associate Dean for Graduate Medical Education, University of Virginia Health System, Charlottesville, Virginia

DILAAWAR J. MISTRY, MD, MS, ATC
Associate Professor of Physical Medicine and Rehabilitation; Internal Medicine Co-Medical Director and Primary Care Team Physician, UVA Sports Medicine, University of Virginia Health System, Charlottesville, Virginia

AUTHORS

SIDDHARTHA S. ANGADI, B.O.Th
Department of Exercise and Wellness, Arizona State University, Mesa, Arizona

EUGENE J. BARRETT, MD, PhD
Professor, Department of Medicine, School of Medicine, University of Virginia, Charlottesville, Virginia

MICHAEL E. CHANSKY, MD
Associate Professor of Emergency Medicine and Internal Medicine, UMDNJ/Robert Wood Johnson Medical School; Chairman, Department of Emergency Medicine, Cooper University Hospital, Camden, New Jersey

MICHAEL CICCHETTI, MD
Resident Physician, Department of Physical Medicine and Rehabilitation, University of Virginia, Charlottesville, Virginia

JILLIAN G. CORBETT, MD
Department of Emergency Medicine, Cooper University Hospital, Camden, New Jersey; Chief Resident and Senior Resident, Emergency Medicine, UMDNJ/Robert Wood Johnson Medical School

EVAN COHEN, MD
Department of Emergency Medicine, Cooper University Hospital, Camden, New Jersey; Junior Resident, Emergency Medicine, UMDNJ/Robert Wood Johnson Medical School

MARK D. DeBOER, MD, MSc, MCR
Assistant Professor of Pediatrics, Department of Pediatrics, Division of Pediatric Endocrinology, University of Virginia School of Medicine, Charlottesville, Virginia

GLENN A. GAESSER, PhD
Department of Exercise and Wellness, Arizona State University, Mesa, Arizona

VIOLA HOLMES, RD, MS
Clinical Nutritionist, Diabetes Education and Management Program, University of Virginia Health System, Charlottesville, Virginia

SUSAN E. KIRK, MD
Associate Professor of Internal Medicine and Obstetrics and Gynecology, Division of Endocrinology and Metabolism; Associate Dean for Graduate Medical Education, University of Virginia Health System, Charlottesville, Virginia

DAVID C. LIEB, MD
Fellow, Department of Medicine, Division of Endocrinology, University of Virginia School of Medicine, Charlottesville, Virginia

JOHN M. MacKNIGHT, MD
Associate Professor, Clinical Internal Medicine and Orthopaedic Surgery; Co-Medical Director for Sports Medicine and Primary Care Team Physician, University of Virginia Health System, Charlottesville, Virginia

ANTHONY McCALL, MD, PhD
Professor of Medicine, Endocrinology and Metabolism, Division of Endocrinology, Department of Internal Medicine, University of Virginia Health System, Charlottesville, Virginia

DILAAWAR J. MISTRY, MD, MS, ATC
Associate Professor of Physical Medicine and Rehabilitation; Internal Medicine Co-Medical Director and Primary Care Team Physician, UVA Sports Medicine, University of Virginia Health System, Charlottesville, Virginia

JOYCE GREEN PASTORS, RD, MS, CDE
Assistant Professor of Education in Internal Medicine, Virginia Center for Diabetes Professional Education, University of Virginia Health System, Charlottesville, Virginia

RAMONA RAJ, MD
Endocrinology Fellow, Division of Endocrinology, Department of Internal Medicine, University of Virginia Health System, Charlottesville, Virginia

COREY A. RYNDERS, BA
Doctoral Student, Department of Human Services, University of Virginia, Charlottesville, Virginia

SUSAN A. SALIBA, PhD, PT, ATC
Assistant Professor, Department of Human Services, Curry School of Education, University of Virginia, Charlottesville, Virginia

RODNEY E. SNOW, MD
Fellow, Department of Medicine, Division of Endocrinology, University of Virginia School of Medicine, Charlottesville, Virginia

ARTHUR WELTMAN, PhD, FACSM
Professor of Human Services, Curry School of Education; Professor of Medicine, School of Medicine, University of Virginia, Charlottesville, Virginia

NATHAN Y. WELTMAN, Med
Physician Scientist Program, Sanford School of Medicine, University of South Dakota, Vermillion, South Dakota

ROBERT P. WILDER, MD, FACSM
Associate Professor, Department of Physical Medicine and Rehabilitation, University of Virginia, Charlottesville, Virginia

Contents

> Pediatric obesity has reached critical proportions. Although this pandemic touches individuals from all socioeconomic, racial, and ethnic backgrounds, the trend is more prevalent among children from families of lower-socioeconomic classes. The causes of this separation in obesity rates by socioeconomic background are multifold but include differences in the availability of healthier foods in homes and schools, as well as the availability of safe environments for physical activity. Equally concerning are increases in the diagnosis of type 2 diabetes among certain ethnic groups and discrepancies in health care availability to children of lower-socioeconomic backgrounds. As our society attempts to improve the lifestyle of our children and decrease rates of obesity, it will be important to give focus to children of lower socioeconomic backgrounds in planning these potential interventions.

> Coronary heart disease is a major cause of morbidity and mortality in persons with diabetes mellitus. Exercise is an important cornerstone in the treatment and management of diabetes but is also associated with a heightened risk of sudden cardiac death in those with occult coronary heart disease. Before beginning a physical activity program that involves anything greater than moderate intensity exercise, consideration should be given to screening asymptomatic persons with diabetes for silent myocardial ischemia.

> As rates of obesity and type 2 diabetes continue to escalate, effective means of prevention become paramount in curbing the largest epidemic of our times. With adult obesity rates in the United States already at 34%, according to the most recent National Health and Nutrition

Examination Survey (NHANES) data, preventing obesity in childhood is of increasing urgency. Exercise and lifestyle modification have been shown to be effective in adult trials for diabetes prevention, such as the Diabetes Prevention Program (DPP), Finnish Diabetes Study, and Da Qing Study. This article reviews randomized, controlled trials in children, using exercise and lifestyle modification in the prevention of insulin resistance and obesity. This review encompasses studies within the past decade from Planet Health in 1999 to the Beijing Obesity Intervention trial published in 2007 and covers both school-based and family-based approaches. A challenging task by any means, these trials have contributed valuable insight into the efficacy of various approaches toward preventing childhood obesity and insulin resistance, a pressing public health concern.

Management of diabetes requires a multidisciplinary approach including: medical therapy, nutritional therapy, self-management education, psychosocial assessment and care, hypoglycemia awareness training, and exercise. Exercise in an effective lifestyle management technique for the prevention of type 2 diabetes and for the management of both type 1 diabetes and type 2 diabetes. Here we review the use of exercise evaluation and prescription for the prevention and management of diabetes.

Musculoskeletal injuries and diseases are common in persons with obesity and diabetes mellitus. High body mass index is associated with an increased risk for musculoskeletal injuries, diseases, and disability. There is a significant positive correlation between the level of obesity and musculoskeletal injuries, and disability and health-related costs. The prevalence of obesity and diabetes is inversely proportional to health-related quality of life.

For many years, one of the mainstays of therapy for patients with either type 1 or type 2 diabetes has been exercise, balanced with medical nutrition therapy and medications. A key limitation to achieving this balance has been the increased risk of hypoglycemia, including that induced by increased glucose use brought about by exercise or athletic activity. This review focuses primarily on type 1 diabetes and athletic activity; however, many of the principles discussed below apply to type 2 diabetes as well.

Diabetes Mellitus is a chronic disorder affecting many adolescents and young adults participating in athletic activity at various levels. If blood glucose levels are managed incorrectly during periods of exercise, diabetes mellitus can lead to various endocrine emergencies, including hypoglycemia, hyperglycemia, and most seriously diabetic ketoacidosis. This article will review the epidemiology of diabetes mellitus, the body's response to exercise in a non-diabetic versus a diabetic, and the pathophysiology, clinical features, treatment, and prevention of hyperglycemic emergencies in athletes.

The unique demands of exercise and competition can predispose diabetic athletes to harmful complications. A basic understanding of glucose metabolism during exercise, nutritional adequacy, blood glucose control, medications, and management of on-field complications is important for medical personnel who care for diabetic athletes on a daily basis. Diabetic athletes are best managed by "individualized" preventive and treatment algorithms that should be developed by a team of medical professionals including the athletic trainer, sports nutritionist, and physician.

THE CLINICS ARE NOW AVAILABLE ONLINE!

Access your subscription at:
www.theclinics.com

Foreword

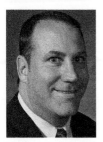

Mark D. Miller, MD
Consulting Editor

It is indeed an honor and a pleasure to introduce this edition of *Clinics in Sports Medicine*. This unique issue focuses on obesity and diabetes and is the result of a coordinated cooperative effort of two of my colleagues at the University of Virginia (UVA). Dr. Mistry and Dr. Kirk are ideally suited to edit this edition. Dr. Mistry is a team physician and co-medical director, and Dr. Kirk is an expert in diabetes in pregnancy and athletes and associate dean of Graduate Medical Education at UVA. Both are associate professors at UVA and are intimately familiar with this topic.

For the orthopods out there, obesity and diabetes are related, and there has been an unfortunate increase in both in our video-gaming, techno-loving, adolescent population. This issue begins with an evaluation of socioeconomic factors in obesity and diabetes. This is followed by a treatise on cardiology screening and 2 articles on exercise in this population. A discussion of common injuries, hypoglycemia, and diabetic emergencies follows. The issue concludes with a practical guide on daily management of athletes with diabetes.

This issue is well written, timely, and of interest to us all. I wish to thank the coeditors, who have done a masterful job in putting this together. Let us recognize and work to solve these problems in our young athletes together!

Mark D. Miller, MD
Division of Sports Medicine
University of Virginia
400 Ray C. Hunt Drive, Suite 330
Charlottesville, VA 22908-0159, USA

E-mail address:
mdm3p@virgina.edu (M.D. Miller)

Clin Sports Med 28 (2009) xi
doi:10.1016/j.csm.2009.03.003
0278-5919/09/$ – see front matter © 2009 Elsevier Inc. All rights reserved.

sportsmed.theclinics.com

Preface

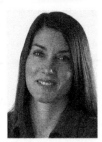 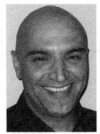

Susan E. Kirk, MD   Dilaawar J. Mistry, MD, MS, ATC
Guest Editors

It is a privilege to contribute to this timely edition of *Clinics of Sports Medicine*. The burden that obesity and diabetes place on society, both in terms of financial cost as well as personal loss, is increasing beyond prediction. This is especially true among our children and adolescents, in whom both obesity and diabetes are epidemic.

Yet there are tremendous disparities when considering these issues in sports medicine. Some athletes with diabetes can, and do, compete at the most elite level. Remember Bobby Clarke from the National Hockey League or Gary Hall, Jr., from the United States Olympic Swim Team? Alternatively, think of current athletes Scott Verplank of the PGA, Jay Cutler of the National Football League, or Adam Morrison of the National Basketball Association. To understand the intricacies of glucose utilization and insulin kinetics, it is essential to develop management strategies that allow these athletes, and thousands more who play in college or high school, to compete at the highest level. Yet, diabetes and obesity are most prevalent in those members of our society who are not at all athletic. Most are sedentary and at considerable risk for cardiovascular diseases. For this population, strategies that increase activities of all types or that emphasize the importance of healthy nutrition are essential. The articles written for this edition span the entire spectrum of these complicated issues. Being able to recognize and treat both the collegiate athlete with type 1 diabetes as well as the sedentary, obese adolescent at risk for type 2 diabetes are skills that many will need in the immediate future.

We truly appreciate the efforts of our fellow authors in contributing to this important issue of *Clinics in Sports Medicine*. Together they have created a composite review that will be valuable to all those who address diabetes and sports: orthopedists and sports medicine specialists, athletic trainers and medical sociologists, and endocrinologists

Clin Sports Med 28 (2009) xiii–xiv
doi:10.1016/j.csm.2009.03.002   **sportsmed.theclinics.com**

and general practitioners. Diabetes and obesity threaten the collective health of our country. We must strive to not only halt but also to reverse this dangerous trend.

Susan E. Kirk, MD
Division of Endocrinology and Metabolism
University of Virginia Health System
McKim Hall, Room 4012
Charlottesville, VA 22908, USA

Dilaawar J. Mistry, MD, MS, ATC
UVA Sports Medicine
University of Virginia Health System
545 Ray C Hunt Drive, Suite 240
Charlottesville, VA 22908, USA

E-mail addresses:
sek4b@virginia.edu (S.E. Kirk)
DM5F@hscmail.mcc.virginia.edu (D.J. Mistry)

Socioeconomic Factors in the Development of Childhood Obesity and Diabetes

David C. Lieb, MD[a], Rodney E. Snow, MD[a],
Mark D. DeBoer, MD, MSc, MCR[b],*

KEYWORDS

• Obesity • Diabetes • Childhood • Socioeconomic disparities
• Physical activity • Nutrition

The pandemic of obesity in the United States has been well publicized through scientific investigation and media reports. Among children in the United States aged 2 to 19 years, 32% are overweight or obese, with body mass indices (BMI) that are above the 85th percentile for age.[1] This increase in obesity has led to an increase in comorbidities, such as hyperlipidemia,[2,3] high blood pressure,[4,5] glucose intolerance,[6,7] type 2 diabetes,[8,9] and evidence of fatty liver disease.[10] If current trends hold out, the generation represented by children born since 2000 is estimated to have a 35% chance of developing diabetes and represents the first generation in the United States since the Civil War to have a life expectancy shorter than that of their parents.[11] As seen in **Fig. 1**, these changes in obesity have been relatively sudden—over the past 20 years—as detrimental changes in lifestyle have become more prevalent in our society. These changes have resulted in lives that have less physical activity and larger quantities of unhealthy foods than ever present previously.

Thus far, our awareness of the problem in children has not helped to turn the tide to begin reversing these trends.[1] Equally disturbing, however, is that in many respects, many of the lifestyle changes in our society that have fueled this epidemic have disproportionately affected children from lower-socioeconomic backgrounds. Many of these increases in obesity have also adversely affected certain racial/ethnic groups more than others. Based on data from the National Health and Nutrition Examination Survey (NHANES) (1976–2002), obesity rates for white, African American, and Mexican

[a] Department of Medicine, Division of Endocrinology, University of Virginia School of Medicine, PO Box 800793, Charlottesville, VA 22908, USA
[b] Department of Pediatrics, Division of Pediatric Endocrinology, University of Virginia School of Medicine, PO Box 800386, Charlottesville, VA 22908, USA
* Corresponding author. PO Box 800386, Charlottesville, VA 22908.
E-mail address: deboer@virginia.edu (M.D. DeBoer).

Clin Sports Med 28 (2009) 349–378
doi:10.1016/j.csm.2009.02.004
0278-5919/09/$ – see front matter © 2009 Elsevier Inc. All rights reserved.

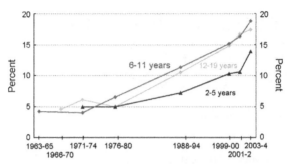

Fig. 1. Trends in childhood and adolescent obesity. Percentage of US children with a BMI ≥ 95th percentile on the 2000 CDC growth charts. (*From* National Health Examination Surveys (NHANES) II (ages 6–11) and III (ages 12–17), NHANES I, II, III and 1999–2004, National Center for Health Statistics, Centers for Disease Control and Prevention.)

American boys and girls (2 to 17 years old) have all increased, but the highest rates were among Mexican American boys and African American girls. Further analyses based on socioeconomic status (SES) of 2- to 19-year-old children from NHANES surveys found higher rates of obesity among all lower-income children. This is seen in **Fig. 2** from a school survey of weight as related to SES level and is further supported by multiple examples of specific societal differences outlined in this review.[12,13]

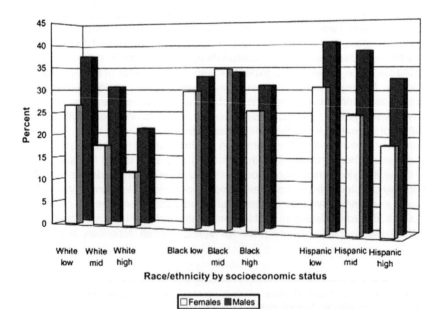

Fig. 2. Childhood overweight compared with socioeconomic standing. Percentage of students at or above the 85th percentile for BMI, eighth and tenth grades, by race/ethnicity and SES for boys (*dark bars*) and girls (*light bars*). Socioeconomic status was determined by reported level of parental education. (*From* Delva J, Johnston LD, O'Malley PM. The epidemiology of overweight and related lifestyle behaviors: racial/ethnic and socioeconomic status differences among American youth. Am J Prev Med 2007;33(4 Suppl):S178–86; with permission.)

Although many of these discrepancies in obesity have been studied specifically along measures of family income, parental education, and other socioeconomic lines, other clear socioeconomic separations are more difficult to discern from the literature. The majority of studies reporting differences in obesity-related lifestyle issues have separated children into racial and ethnic groups (eg, white, African American, and Hispanic). Although this method of dividing groups of children does not necessarily reflect social or economic divisions, for the sake of this review, we present the racial/ethnicity data alongside more reliable socioeconomic data, acknowledging that the racial/ethnicity data may not completely represent socioeconomic differences but offers the best glimpse that we can obtain from the current literature.

It is important to examine these socioeconomic factors as they pertain to patterns of lifestyle, obesity, and diabetes, because as our society faces the need to recreate a more healthy lifestyle in our populations, we will need to be mindful to concentrate efforts on lower-socioeconomic groups that may have greater needs for change but less means to afford the associated costs. These costs are related to alterations in eating patterns and physical activity, each of which has contributed to worsened rates of childhood obesity and diabetes as well as to the widening differences between SES groups. We additionally consider differences in the care for type 2 diabetes as well as targeted solutions to bridge these gaps.

SOCIOECONOMIC DISCREPANCIES IN NUTRITION
Shifts in the US Food Environment

A major root cause of the worsening rates of obesity in the United States relates to changes in the eating habits of Americans. The food environment that children in the United States are exposed to changed dramatically during the twentieth century. This altered nutritional environment, coupled with decreased physical activity, contributed to a cumulative energy imbalance, leading to a rise in adult and pediatric obesity. The differences in the food environment in the United States today compared with that in the mid-twentieth century are the result of fundamental changes in food characteristics, such as quality, quantity, and availability. Consistent with the theme of this article, epidemiologic studies have demonstrated that the impact of these changes on the food environment have been more significant for middle- and lower-SES families.

Alterations to food characteristics have included increased energy density,[14] portion sizes,[15] and variety,[16] all of which have been shown in controlled studies to increase total energy intake at meals. The persistence of these modifications to the food environment has been shown to override physiologic regulatory systems and exert more long-term effects on human energy regulation than were previously estimated.[17] Similarly, consistent increases in energy intake have been effectively demonstrated in children who were given successively larger portions of food.[17] This new food environment, rich in a variety of processed foods (with added sugar and fat), followed by progressively larger portions, has allowed for an excessive and unbalanced intake of energy and nutrients.[18] Although children of all ages, gender, race, and SES are currently exposed to this new environment, there is a persistent gap in obesity rates between ethnic minorities and lower-SES children and adolescents compared with their white or more affluent counterparts.[19]

Socioeconomic Differences in Obesity Rates

Geographically, the estimated prevalence of obesity in adults ($\geq$20 years old) in 2006 ranged from 18.7% to 31.9% between states and as much as 9.8% to 36.9% between

US counties.[20] The geographic distributions of adult and pediatric obesity suggest additional environmental influences on food intake, such as the social and economic characteristics of different regions in the United States.[21,22] Furthermore, as the era of cheap, abundant, and calorie-dense food emerged, obesity became clinically apparent nation-wide in men, women, and children across all socioeconomic levels, but the degree of obesity was shown to vary by race, gender, income, education, and location.

For adults (≥20 years old), the degree of obesity by race/ethnicity has been highest in African American women (53.9%) followed by Hispanic women (42.3%) and African American men (34%). In comparison, obesity rates for white women and men were 30.2 and 31.1%, respectively.[23] Compared with males, females have shown consistently larger inverse associations with obesity and income since 1970, most notably in African American and white women.[24] In a study of nearly 7,000 US citizens, statistically significant increases in obesity rates were shown in lower-income (less than 130% of federal poverty line) and lower-education households (less than high school).[25]

For adolescents, similar geographic disparities were recently described in a study sampling 46,707 children aged 10 to 17 years across the United States and District of Columbia. For regional and state disparities, the strongest association with adolescent obesity was found in household incomes below the poverty level.[25] However, the association between family income and childhood obesity has been shown to vary by race, because income was positively associated with BMI in African American children and negatively associated with BMI in white children.[26]

Changes in Food as a Cause of Worsening Obesity

Multiple trends in food availability over the past 50 years have contributed to our current predicament. Before the 1970s, the food industry was already adapting to meet increasing demands for convenient foods by a post-World War II work force increasingly populated by working mothers and the subsequent rise of "2-income" families. Between 1960 and 2005, female labor force activity rose at every level of education, but participation rates differed according to race and income of the spouse (**Fig. 3**). By 2005, 65% of married African American mothers worked compared with

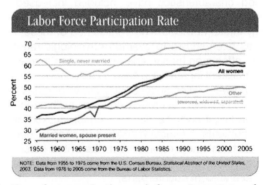

Fig. 3. The participation of women in the work force. Percentage of married and single women working in the United States by year. (*From* Engemann KM, Owyang MT. Social Changes Lead Married Women into Labor Force. The Regional Economist. A Quarterly Review of Business and Economic Conditions. The Federal Reserve Bank of St. Louis. April 2006; with permission.)

58% of white, 51% Asian, and 34% of Hispanic mothers. Overall, household income data show that work-force participation has been highest for working mothers whose husbands were in the middle-earnings quintile. However, since 1997, participation rates for all white mothers fell by 4.5%, regardless of spouse income, whereas rates for African American mothers whose husbands were in the lowest quintile of earnings held steady.[27] The assumption here is that nutritious meals at home take more time and money to purchase and prepare, and families with lower incomes and less time spent at home depend more on precooked and convenient foods, which are energy dense.

Dramatic increases in the supply of US food commodities have occurred in response to the significant food-price inflation of the early 1970s. This inflation led to an abundance of cheaper substrates (corn, soybeans) from which a new era of highly processed foods with higher fat and sugar content have emerged. These surpluses, coupled with food science technology, fueled the exponential increase of new, inexpensive, processed foods throughout the 1980s. Although these additives have not been proven to directly cause obesity, the effects of increased availability and aggressive marketing of these new products on human consumption are clear.

The industry of food and beverage sales is a narrow-profit-margin business, and as the variety of food products expanded, the competition for each food dollar of the US consumer increased.[28] Eventually, food manufacturers realized that children were more than just passive recipients of the foods their parents chose. Instead, children were increasingly seen as consumers, with growing independence and significant influence over the purchasing choices of adults. By 1999, children aged 6 to 19 years were estimated to have influenced $485 billion in purchasing decisions each year.[29] Although not proven to directly cause childhood obesity, there is a clear "time-course" association between childhood obesity and the increased availability of calorie-dense processed foods, which are marketed directly to children (**Fig. 4**).[16] The amount of

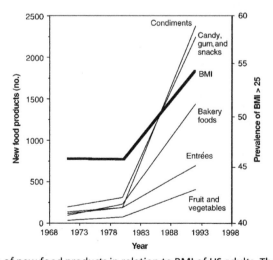

Fig. 4. Emergence of new food products in relation to BMI of US adults. The number of new, calorie-dense food products introduced to the US market has paralleled the rise in obesity, whereas introduction of new fruits and vegetable products was dramatically less during the same period. (*From* McCrory MA, Fuss PJ, McCallum JE, et al. Dietary variety within food groups: association with energy intake and body fatness in men and women. Am J Clin Nutr 1999;69(3):440–7; with permission.)

advertising money spent on all marketing to children rose from $6.9 billion (1992) to $12.7 billion (1997),[28] whereas consumption of fat and carbohydrates increased in children (aged 11–18 years) by 4% and 15%, and obesity rates in this age group tripled from 1980 to 2006.[30] A 2004 study found that food-related (TV) advertising made up 26% of advertised products viewed by adolescents, and the proportion of exposure to these advertisements were 14% greater for African American versus white adolescents aged 12 to 17 years.[31] Potential explanations for this difference were higher TV viewing rates in this population, with marketing campaigns targeting them specifically.

Although the marketing of energy-dense, processed foods has been ubiquitous, availability of these processed foods in relation to healthier options has been demonstrated to differ among neighborhoods and according to SES. Regarding the food eaten at home, most families obtain their foods from the nearest grocery store. However, grocery stores across the country have been shown to differ in quality and prices of foods offered. Supermarkets have been shown to be more likely to stock healthful foods at a lower cost than smaller grocery stores. Study results based on multistate samples have found that low- versus high-income neighborhoods and predominantly black versus white neighborhoods have fewer numbers of available supermarkets but significantly more grocery and convenience stores and thus a lower proportion of healthier options for customers.[21] Furthermore, low-income families with proportionally higher costs of living have less money for food, which encourages a propensity for inexpensive but high-calorie foods.[32]

Food Away from Home

The percent of total income spent on food away from home increased from 26% in 1970 to 39% by 1996.[33] Factors cited to contribute to this growing trend of dining out are the rise of 2-income households, higher incomes, less expensive but more convenient fast food, smaller family size, and pervasive advertising of food-service establishments.[34] Between 1977 and 1996, American families increased the proportion of total energy obtained from restaurants and fast-food establishments and decreased the proportion of that obtained from home. Between 1977 and 1996, children ages 2 to 18 years decreased their total percent of energy eaten at home by 10.5% (75.7%–65.2%), increased the percentage of energy obtained from restaurant/fast food by 10% (4.8%–14.8%), and decreased total energy intake from school by 2.2%. Thus, it is not surprising that energy intake from restaurant/fast food increased by between 91.2% and 208% for all age groups.[35]

With regard to children in the United States, perhaps the most influential food-service establishment is the US public school system. Children spend approximately 8 h/d and 180 days/y on school property. Over 25 million students use the National School Lunch Program (NSLP) daily, whereas approximately 7 million use the National School Breakfast Program (NSBP) daily.[36] Meals from these programs may constitute more than half the daily caloric intake for children who participate in both programs, particularly for those from low-income families. Due to the fact that pediatric obesity is more prevalent in lower socioeconomic groups, such children from these groups may be influenced more significantly by the content of these free or discounted meals.[37]

Over the past 4 decades, local budgetary changes began forcing schools to move the preparation of school meals to off-site locations, thus relinquishing the nutritional control over cafeteria meals once held by on-site food preparation staff.[38] Eventually, the traditional school cafeteria has transformed from an adequately funded, large-scale kitchen where food is prepared by skilled staff to merely a final site of assembly for precooked food products that require minimally trained staff. As a result, according to a 2007 US Department of Agriculture (USDA) report, less than one-third of US public schools were able to meet the recommended standard for either total or saturated fat in their meals.[39]

Another factor contributing to pediatric obesity is the emergence of direct marketing and sale of food to children inside schools but outside of federal school lunch programs. Consistent budget shortfalls have created an environment increasingly open to entrepreneurial opportunities. In the early 1990s, fast-food companies began selling products directly to school children by posting kiosks outside of school cafeterias, thus avoiding long-standing federal restrictions on such foods inside school cafeterias. School districts generated revenues by purchasing discounted fast-food products and marking them up before sale to school children.[38] For poorer school districts, this meant increased revenues by allowing fast-food companies to "establish their brand" inside schools.[40]

Soft drinks have been sold in schools since the 1960s, predominantly through vending machines in teachers' lounges and as concessions at sporting events. By the mid-1990s, a more symbiotic relationship began to emerge between schools and soft-drink companies. In the early 1990s, large soft-drink companies began offering exclusive "pouring rights" contracts to school districts that included elementary-, middle-, and high school facilities. These contracts were similar to the arrangements between a soda manufacturer and University stadiums and entailed 3 monetary payments for 3 contractual promises. First, in return for exclusively selling 1 brand of soda, schools would receive commissions and yearly bonus payments, both of which were tied to the quantity of sodas sold. Second, schools would receive free product to sell at fund-raising events if they agreed to display that brand's advertising on campus.[28] Third, companies offered more aid to school fund-raising events if their products were available during all school hours.[38] Between 1985 and 1997, soda sales to US schools increased 1100%, whereas milk sales to schools declined 30%.[28] By 2005, 67% of middle and 83% of US high school students were enrolled in schools with some form of a "pouring contract," with the only SES variance being that Hispanic students were more likely than other ethnicities to have soft drinks available throughout the school day.[40]

Many studies have now shown this significant relationship between children and beverage intake. USDA national survey data indicate that between 1965 and 1996, declining milk intakes were observed, whereas soft-drink and noncitrus juice intake increased in adolescents 11 to 18 years of age.[30] By the year 2000, soft drinks were the leading source of added sugar in the diet and were estimated to contribute 36.2 g and 57.7 g daily to adolescent girls and boys, respectively.[41] In children aged 2 to 17 years participating in the 1994 to 1996 Continuing Survey of Food Intakes by Individuals, milk intake was positively associated with recommended intakes of vitamin A, folate, vitamin B-12, calcium, and mangnesium.[42] In 2005, a study of 645 children aged 1 to 5 years found that milk intake was inversely associated with intakes of juice drinks, sodas, and added-sugar beverages for all age groups.[43] A 2001 prospective, observational study of 548 ethnically diverse school children with an average age of 11.7 years found that for each additional serving of sugar-sweetened drinks, both BMI and frequency of obesity significantly increased (adjusted for anthropometric, demographic, dietary, and lifestyle variables).[44]

The association between an underfunded school environment, likely to provide calorie-dense foods and beverages, and childhood obesity is highlighted by studies showing that school SES and racial/ethnic composition are inversely related to BMI, even after controlling for these factors.[45] Lower income, urban, African American, and Hispanic community rates of childhood overweight or obesity have been documented to be as high as 40% in elementary school populations.[46] Although the environmental factors mentioned here have not been proven to directly cause obesity, the association is undeniable, and broad efforts are being made to remove these influences from all schools in response to the epidemic of childhood and adolescent obesity. For example, Los Angeles County schools have banned sales of soda and snacks at all schools, and efforts in Minnesota schools have introduced programs to increase the amount of fruits and vegetables served, as discussed later in the section "Targeted Approaches to Improving Childhood Nutrition."

SOCIOECONOMICS OF PHYSICAL ACTIVITY IN OBESITY AND DIABETES IN CHILDREN
Physical Activity in Children and Adolescents

Physical activity was once a critical part of daily life for all human beings, young and old. The conveniences of modern life (transportation, easy food sources) and some of the inconveniences (crime, lack of time for engaging in exercise and other healthy behaviors) have changed this considerably. In children and adolescents, this had led to increasing rates of both diabetes and obesity.[47] Multiple factors, including those related to SES, affect a child's level of physical activity and fitness, from the activity level of their parents and friends to the distance they must travel to get to the nearest, safe playground.

Measuring levels of physical activity in children can be difficult, especially in younger children.[47] Many studies rely upon self-reporting, interviews, and questionnaires. Although these are often easier to perform than direct measurements of activity, they are not always accurate.[48] Younger children might not be able to report their activity appropriately, and as with all studies involving self-reporting, the opportunity for recall bias exists. More recent studies have taken advantage of technology, using devices such as accelerometers that provide more objective data.[49] These devices can record periods of activity and provide an estimate of that activity's intensity. Of course, compliance issues can arise with these devices as well.

The American Heart Association, in their 2005 Scientific Statement regarding the prevention and treatment of overweight/obesity in children and adolescents, recommends that children engage in 30 to 60 minutes of regular exercise daily. They define an adequate effort as exercise that causes the participant to "work up a sweat." They also recommend limiting sedentary behaviors to less than 2 h/d.[50] However, how frequently are American children meeting these recommendations? In a longitudinal study of over 1,000 children aged 9 to 15 years, the National Institute of Child Health and Human Development's Study of Early Child Care and Youth Development found that at 9 years of age, children were involved in approximately 3 hours of "moderate-to-vigorous activity" per day (including weekdays and weekends).[51] Investigators found that, each year, the amount of time that participants were involved in moderate-to-vigorous activity declined by approximately 40 minutes. By age 15, participants were exercising for only between 35 and 49 min/d. The decline in time spent active was seen in both boys and girls, though boys remained somewhat more active for a longer period of time (**Fig. 5**).[51] In a similar study using accelerometer data from individuals aged 6 to 20 years and older, Troiano and colleagues reported that activity levels declined significantly between the 6- to 11-year-old age group and those aged 12 to 19 years.[52] They found that although 42% of 6- to 11-year-old children engaged in at least 60 minutes of physical activity daily, only 8% of older children and adolescents did so. They also noted that less than 5% of the adults studied engaged in 30 minutes of exercise daily.

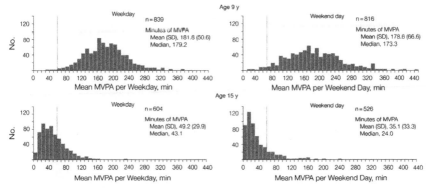

Fig. 5. Decline in physical activity with age. Distribution of time spent performing moderate to vigorous physical activity (MVPA) as measured by accelerometers worn by children aged 9 (*upper graphs*) and 15 (*lower graphs*) years on weekdays and weekends. (*From* Nader PR, Bradley RH, Houts RM, McRitchie SL, O'Brien M. Moderate-to-vigorous physical activity from ages 9 to 15 years. JAMA 2008;300(3):295–305; with permission.)

Decreased Physical Activity and Childhood Obesity

Decreased (or the complete lack of) physical activity is associated with a number of concerning outcomes in children and adolescents. Data from the Centers for Disease Control and Prevention (CDC) Youth Risk Behavior Survey performed in 1999 revealed strong correlations between one's physical activity level and body weight.[53] More than 15,000 US adolescents aged 14 to 18 years were surveyed, and multiple racial groups were represented. Participants were given questionnaires to determine their level of physical activity (either moderate or vigorous) as well as the number of hours they spent watching TV on school days. BMI was significantly lower in those participants engaged in at least moderate physical activity. Conversely, lower levels of physical activity were associated with an increased risk for being overweight. There was a graded correlation between TV watching and being overweight (**Table 1**). Those who watched 4 or more hours of TV per school day were the most likely to be overweight, whereas those reporting less than 1 hour of TV watching per day were approximately 40% less likely to be overweight. Notably, the impact that TV watching had on weight appeared to be more significant than that of physical activity alone.

Studies have shown that a child's degree or severity of obesity correlates with the prevalence of the metabolic syndrome, a condition involving insulin resistance and hyperglycemia that is associated with poor cardiovascular outcomes. A study

Table 1
Association between moderate physical activity, television watching, and overweight status in US boys and girls (ages 14–18)

Group	Moderate Physical Activity		Television Watched	
	<2 d/wk	6–7 d/wk	<1 h/d	>4 h/d
Boys	1.37 (1.17–1.61; P<.001)	1.0	0.58 (0.48–0.71; P<.001)	1.0
Girls	1.10 (0.74–1.65; P = NS)	1.0	0.61 (0.49–0.77; P = .05)	1.0

Data presented as odds ratio with 95% confidence interval, followed by significance (*P* value).
Data from Eisenmann JC, Bartee RT, Wang MQ. Physical activity, TV viewing, and weight in U.S. youth: 1999 Youth Risk Behavior Survey. Obes Res 2002;10(5):379–85.

of overweight and obese children and adolescents by Weiss and colleagues in 2004 found that almost 50% of severely obese children met the criteria for the metabolic syndrome. Biomarkers of increased cardiovascular risk, such as low levels of the protective adipose tissue hormone, adiponectin, and elevated concentrations of C-reactive protein, a marker of potentially harmful inflammation and cardiovascular risk, were seen in these children.[7] Notably, being overweight or obese in childhood predicts an increased risk of being overweight as an adult.[54]

Decreased Physical Activity and Diabetes

Certainly, one of the most concerning consequences of decreased physical activity and increased obesity in children is the development of insulin resistance and diabetes. The incidence of type 2 diabetes in children is increasing.[55,56] Although few, if any, long-term data regarding activity level and risk for diabetes in children and adolescents exist, data are available that demonstrate that sedentary behavior is associated with an increased risk for developing type 2 diabetes in both adult men and women. Hu and colleagues[57] found that the relative risk of developing type 2 diabetes in men in the United States was increased by more than 1.5 times in those who watched between 2 and 10 hours of TV per week compared with those who watched less than 1 hour. Those who watched more than 40 h/wk had a risk of developing diabetes that was almost 3 times that of individuals who watched less than 1 hour weekly. In women, each 2-hour increase in TV watching time per day was associated with a 14% increase in the risk of developing type 2 diabetes (**Table 2**).[58] Each 2-hour daily increase in the amount of time spent sitting at work was associated with an increased risk of 7%. Conversely, 1 hour of walking briskly per day was associated with a 34% reduction in the risk of developing diabetes. The authors estimated that 43% of new cases of type 2 diabetes in women could be prevented by watching less than 10 hours of TV per week and walking briskly for at least 30 minutes daily.

A study of children with type 1 diabetes in Norway found that children who watched more than 4 hours of TV daily had a significantly higher hemoglobin A1c (9.5% ± 1.6) than that of those who watched less than 1 hour of TV daily (mean A1c, 8.2% ± 0.9%).[59] This significant trend remained valid even when adjustments were made for BMI and insulin dose.

Other Effects of Decreased Physical Activity in Children and Adolescents

Physical activity has been associated with an improvement in a child's self-esteem. In fact, some studies have suggested that high-level activity (as defined by a biaxial

Table 2
Relative risk (RR) of having type 2 diabetes according to number of hours of television watched per week in US men and women

Group	Average Number of Hours of Television Watched per Week			
	0–1 h	21–40 h	>40 h	P for Trend
Men (RR), age-adjusted	1.0	2.22 (1.49–3.31)	3.35 (1.71–6.55)	<0.001
Women (RR), age-adjusted	1.0	1.53 (1.19–1.96)	1.98 (1.39–2.81)	<0.001

Data presented as RR with 95% confidence interval.
Data from Hu FB, Leitzmann MF, Stampfer MJ, et al. Physical activity and television watching in relation to risk for type 2 diabetes mellitus in men. Arch Intern Med 2001;161(12):1542–8; and Hu FB, Li TY, Colditz GA, et al. Television watching and other sedentary behaviors in relation to risk of obesity and type 2 diabetes mellitus in women. JAMA 2003;289(14):1785–91.

accelerometer) has a positive effect on improving self-esteem but that moderate-level activity does not.[60] The converse of this is also true—obesity, a major outcome of low levels of physical activity, is correlated with lower levels of self-esteem in children.[61] Studies have also looked at the effect of physical activity on bone density in adolescents. This is an important consideration to make, given that children and adolescents are still growing and building bone strength. The Amsterdam Growth and Health Longitudinal Study found that increased daily physical activity (as determined by subject interviews, with subsequent scores based on frequency, duration, and peak strain of activity reported) correlated positively with lumbar and hipbone mineral density.[62] These subjects included male and female adolescents who were followed from age 13 to age 29 years. Neuromotor fitness, (as defined by a composite score of speed, flexibility, and strength tests, including leg lifts, standing high jump, arm pull, bent arm hang, shuttle run, plate tapping, and sit and reach), but not cardiorespiratory fitness (as defined by maximal oxygen uptake or $Vo_{2\,max}$), correlated positively with bone density. When these individuals were followed though young adulthood (up to age 36 years), the male participants continued to have an improved lumbar bone mineral density when correlated with the mechanical aspects of the activity (sum of all ground forces) but not metabolic aspects of the activity (intensity, duration, and frequency).[63] Female subjects had no correlation between either form of activity and lumbar spine density. The effects that these improvements in bone density will have on fracture risk in later adulthood are less clear.

Low levels of physical activity are associated with other poor health choices and behaviors in children and adolescents. The 1990 Youth Risk Behavior Survey evaluated more than 11,000 high school students throughout the United States. The survey found that adolescents who participated in low activity (fewer than 2 days of "light exercise that made [them] breathe a little more than usual and made [their] heart beat a little faster than usual") over a 2-week period were more likely to smoke cigarettes, eat fewer fruits and vegetables, use marijuana, and not wear a seat belt.[64]

Physical Activity and Minority and Low-Socioeconomic Populations

Previous studies have suggested that particular ethnic minorities are less physically active and less physically fit. Pivarnik and colleagues[65] found that African American adolescent girls had significantly lower aerobic fitness (as assessed by $Vo_{2\,max}$) and were not able to use a treadmill for as long as their white counterparts. Simons-Morton and colleagues[66] reported a study of more than 2,000 third-grade students living in California, Texas, Minnesota, and Louisiana. They found that white students reported significantly more minutes of physical activity than African American or Hispanic students did. However, when multiple factors were included in their analysis (such as geographic location of the participants), ethnicity was no longer associated with lower levels of physical activity.[66] In a study of 107 children (mean age, 10 years) in Birmingham, Alabama, there were no significant differences between white and African American children in the hours of exercise they reported per week or in the number of days per week they exercised.[67] There were also no differences in sports team participation between the 2 ethnic groups. However, African American students spent approximately 40 minutes less time in physical education class at school, for reasons that are unclear. White children also had higher aerobic capacity than that of African American children.

Two large studies have evaluated the differences in physical activity between minority and low-SES children and their peers. The "Monitoring the Future" and "Youth, Education, and Society" studies surveyed almost 54,000 eighth-, tenth-, and twelfth-grade students from across the United States.[68] These surveys found that the percentage of students in schools requiring physical education decreased sharply from 87% among eighth graders to 20% among those in twelfth grade. Of all eighth-grade students, significantly fewer Hispanic students (75.9%) were exposed to physical education than their white peers (89.3%; $P<.05$). However, schools attended by African American and Hispanic students had higher numbers of students walking or biking to school. The surveys also found that children from lower-SES groups (as defined by level of parental education) were less likely to attend schools that required physical education (49.6% for those in the lowest SES group compared with 59.2% for those in the highest). Students from lower-SES groups were also less likely to participate in varsity or intramural sports or physical activity clubs, differences that held true for both boys and girls (**Table 3**). These discrepancies in physical education and activity place those from a lower SES at a great disadvantage, as their decreased physical activity places them at high risk for becoming overweight and obese.[68]

Sedentary Behaviors, Minority Groups, and Low Socioeconomic Status

Children in the United States participate in a number of sedentary behaviors, from TV and movie watching, to playing video games, to reading. Although a controlled amount of these behaviors may be stress reducing and healthy, this can only be the case if these behaviors are not performed at the expense of regular physical activity. As with physical activity, an individual's SES can play an important role in modulating one's risk for developing obesity or diabetes. Data from the NHANES III, which surveyed more than 4,000 American children between 1988 and 1994, showed that 80% of all US children were engaged in at least 3 episodes of vigorous physical activity per week.[69] These rates were lower in Mexican American girls (73%) and non-Hispanic black girls (69%). Girls were, overall, less active than boys (**Table 4**). With regard to their TV viewing habits, one-quarter of all children surveyed watched at least 4 hours of TV daily, and two-thirds watched at least 2 hours daily. About 42% of non-Hispanic black children watched 4 or more hours, and those children who watched more than 4 h/d had a greater BMI and body fat percentage than those who watched less than 2 hours daily.

In a study of British children and adolescents (aged 11–16 years), those from lower-SES neighborhoods were significantly more sedentary than those from higher-SES locales. Boys from lower-SES neighborhoods spent almost 2.5 more hours engaged

Table 3
Physical education school requirement and participation in interscholastic/varsity sports by SES

Variable	Student Socioeconomic Status				
	1 (Low)	2	3	4	5 (High)
% of students for whom PE required	49.6	51.8	50.2	55.2	59.2[a]
% Boys participating in scholastic/varsity sports	31.7	35.9	37.1	39.1	39.7[b]
% Girls participating in scholastic/varsity sports	27.4	31.9	33.0	35.0	35.6[b]

Data presented represent US eight, tenth, and twelfth graders as broken by SES, with 1 being lower SES and 5 being higher SES. Data presented as percentages.
Significance of linear association shown.
[a] $P<0.01$.
[b] $P<0.001$.
Data from Johnston LD, Delva J, O'Malley PM. Sports participation and physical education in American secondary schools: current levels and racial/ethnic and socioeconomic disparities. Am J Prev Med 2007;33(4 Suppl):S195–208.

Table 4
Unadjusted prevalence of number of weekly sessions of vigorous play or exercise in US youth (aged 8–16 y)

Group (Aged 8–16 y)	Prevalence of Reported Sessions per Week of Vigorous Play/Exercise		
	≤1 Session	2 Sessions	≥3 Sessions
Non-Hispanic white			
Boys	3.4	8.8	87.9
Girls	10.9	12.0	77.1
Non-Hispanic black			
Boys	9.4	13.0	77.6
Girls	15.8	14.8	69.4
Mexican American			
Boys	7.4	12.4	80.2
Girls	15.4	11.9	72.6

Data presented as prevalence (per 100%).
Data from Andersen RE, Crespo CJ, Bartlett SJ, et al. Relationship of physical activity and television watching with body weight and level of fatness among children: results from the Third National Health and Nutrition Examination Survey. JAMA 1998;279(12):938–42.

in sedentary behavior each week than their peers, and girls spent more than 4 more hours per week.[70]

Interestingly, some of the traditionally sedentary behaviors in which children and adolescents engage are becoming more active. The popularity of the Nintendo Wii home entertainment system is one such example. Of course, the energy expended while using such a system does not equal that of actually playing sports.[71] Furthermore, these systems are expensive, and may not be available to children from lower socioeconomic backgrounds. However, the addition of the concept of "active" play with activities typically associated with purely sedentary behavior is a step in the right direction.

Community Resources, Crime, and Physical Activity

The community in which a child lives can have a great effect on his or her level of physical activity. Gordon-Larsen and colleagues[72] studied a group of more than 20,000 American adolescents in a variety of community types between 1994 and 1995. They found that communities with more college-educated individuals had a wider variety and number of facilities available for physical activity than communities with a lower-educated populace. Furthermore, as the minority population in an area increased, the odds of having any physical fitness facility at all decreased. Communities with more facilities available had more active adolescents, and subsequently, lower numbers of overweight individuals. Adolescents who lived in areas with at least 7 facilities available for exercise and physical activity were 26% more likely to be active than those who lived in areas without any facilities and were 32% less likely to be overweight.

The perceived level of crime in a neighborhood is often another deterrent to physical activity in a community. One study that looked into this issue involved the Behavioral Risk Factor Surveillance System, a telephone survey of individuals at least 18 years of age in Maryland, Ohio, Virginia, Pennsylvania, and Montana.[73] Those surveyed were asked to report how safe they felt in their neighborhood and were also asked about their own physical activity. About 30% of respondents indicated that they were physically inactive. Inactivity was increased in older adults, ethnic minorities, those with less education, and in those with annual household incomes less than $ 20,000 dollars. In this study, the *perceived* degree of safety in one's neighborhood was associated with the degree of physical activity in which that individual was involved, though the study did not report the actual crime levels in the neighborhoods. Studies have also shown that women, and particularly women from minority groups, are hesitant to use public spaces for physical activity given concerns for their safety.[74] Furthermore, the parents of ethnic minority children are often hesitant to allow their children to engage in after-school activities and report concern for safe travel to and from the activities as one reason for their concern.[74] A study of the mothers of more than 3,000 3-year-old children in twenty large cities in the United States found that maternal perception of neighborhood safety was not associated with decreased weekday or weekend outdoor playtime. However, those children living in the neighborhoods perceived to be the least safe spent the most amount of time indoors watching TV.[75] Another study surveying fourth-grade children found that although children from low socioeconomic backgrounds found more "hazards" in their neighborhoods (including crime, gangs, drugs, prejudice, traffic, trash and litter, among other items), they reported higher levels of physical activity than children from higher-socioeconomic families.[76] The reasons for these discrepancies are unclear.

A child's parents and friends may have a significant effect on the child's activity level and the amount of sedentary behavior in which he or she takes part. A study of adolescents in Norway (mean age, 13.3 years) found that individuals with parents and friends who valued physical activity and helped engage the adolescent in some form of activity were more likely to be physically active themselves.[77] An 8-year-long study from the same group, however, found that there were only weak associations between the physical activity levels of parents and their children.[77] The previously discussed study of children in Birmingham, Alabama, found that children in a single-parent home spent significantly more time watching TV than those in a dual-parent home and also spent less time exercising in physical education classes at school.[67] Ethnicity and gender were not associated with higher TV watching. It is worth noting that children from single-parent homes exercised more days per week than their counterparts do and also had higher levels of aerobic fitness (as measured by $Vo_{2\ max}$).[67] These studies demonstrate the complexity with which one's social environment affects the ability to engage in regular physical activity and, thus, improve the risk factors for obesity and diabetes.

American children and adolescents are less active than they were in the past, and as a result are more overweight and obese, and have complications of obesity such as diabetes. There are multiple reasons for this decrease in physical activity. Some are more obvious, such as large amounts of sedentary behavior, including TV watching. Other factors such as the communities in which children live and their socioeconomic circumstances are more complex. Further studies are needed to gain a better understanding of the barriers children face when attempting to become more physically active.

SOCIOECONOMICS OF DIABETES IN CHILDREN

Many people are aware of the global obesity epidemic affecting children and adolescents. However, fewer people realize the toll that poor food choices and sedentary behavior have had on another growing problem affecting children—diabetes. As with obesity, those from lower socioeconomic backgrounds have abundant barriers to overcome when approaching this dangerous disease. Though touched on already in this review, the section that follows provides greater detail regarding diabetes in children and adolescents. It first describes this growing problem in terms of increasing prevalence and incidence and then details the difficulties that minority groups and those from a lower socioeconomic background face with regard to both disease burden and management.

Prevalence and Incidence of Diabetes in Children

Diabetes is a complex and costly medical condition affecting millions of people worldwide and is one of the major medical consequences of the obesity epidemic. According to data from the NHANES conducted between 1999 and 2002, the prevalence of diabetes (diagnosed and undiagnosed) in the United States was 9.3% of the population or 19.3 million Americans.[78] This number has increased significantly from a prevalence of 7.8% between 1988 and 1994. Importantly, the 1999 to 2002 data showed that African Americans and Mexican Americans had twice the prevalence of that in non-Hispanic whites. The most recent data available from the CDC indicate that 23.6 million Americans aged 20 years and older have diabetes (both diagnosed and undiagnosed). Interestingly, this equates to a prevalence of 7.8%, indicating that the overall prevalence of diabetes in the United States may have decreased since the earlier NHANES report.[79] The increase in diabetes is a global problem, with the World Health Organization estimating that the global prevalence of diabetes will increase from 2.8% in 2004 to 4.4% by 2030. This equates to 366 million people living with diabetes.[80] No population is spared—all races, socioeconomic groups, and ages are affected by this disease, though certain ethnic groups appear to be more affected than others. For example, although children born in the United States in 2000 are estimated to have more than a 30% chance of developing diabetes in their lifetime, this estimate increases to 52.5% among Hispanic females.[11]

When determining the prevalence and incidence of diabetes in children and adolescents, one must first define the type of diabetes that is being evaluated. Although type 2 diabetes is more closely associated with the obesity epidemic and socioeconomic discrepancies, type 1 diabetes remains more prevalent among children, comprising at least 80% of children with diabetes. Type 1 diabetes is typically associated with autoimmunity (positive antibodies) and severely decreased or the complete lack of insulin production.[81] Although some studies have suggested a role for various socioeconomic factors (smaller family size, increased family income) in the pathogenesis of type 1 diabetes, others have shown no clear association between SES and this form of the disease.[82]

Type 2 diabetes was once considered a disease of adulthood, but as children and adolescents have become more overweight and obese, type 2 diabetes has become much more common in this younger generation. Case series performed in major US cities in the 1990s showed that, depending on the community, 8% to 45% of newly diagnosed cases of diabetes in individuals aged 19 years or younger were type 2 diabetes (**Table 5**).[83] These studies included children of various ethnic backgrounds, including whites, African Americans, and Hispanics.

One report from a registry in New York found that during a 10-year period, the number of patients younger than 18 years of age with type 2 diabetes increased by a factor of 10.[56] Another case series studying newly diagnosed diabetic adolescents in Cincinnati found that the incidence of noninsulin-dependent diabetes in that population had increased from 0.7/100,000/y in 1982 to 7.2/100,000/y in 1994.[55]

Most children with type 2 diabetes are overweight or obese, with case series reporting mean BMI estimates ranging from 27 to 38 kg/m^2.[84,85] In a study of 167 obese children and adolescents, Sinha and colleagues[6] found that between 21% and 25% had

Table 5
New cases of type 2 diabetes in US children and adolescents, 1982–1997

Study	Race/Ethnicity	Age (y)	Estimated % of New Cases
San Diego, CA	W, AA, H, AsA	0–16	8
Cincinnati, OH	W, AA	0–19	16
		10–19	33
San Antonio, TX	W, H		18
Ventura, CA	H	0–17	45

Studies include case series only. Data presented as estimated percentage of cases of type 2 diabetes out of all newly diagnosed cases of diabetes.
Abbreviations: W, Whites; AA, African Americans; H, Hispanics; AsA, Asian Americans.
Data from American Diabetes Association. Type 2 diabetes in children and adolescents. Diabetes Care 2000;23(3):381–9.

impaired glucose tolerance, a precursor to developing diabetes, and that 4% had undiagnosed type 2 diabetes. Therefore, as the number of obese children increases in the United States and in other countries, the incidence of new cases of type 2 diabetes will increase concomitantly. It should be noted that as the obesity epidemic in children in the United States continues, many type 1 diabetics will become overweight or obese, and, subsequently, insulin-resistant as well.[86] These individuals may, then, have a similar risk for cardiovascular disease as those children and adolescents with type 2 diabetes. Research has suggested that insulin resistance in type 1 diabetic patients is associated with an increased risk for cardiovascular morbidity and mortality. Ten-year follow-up from the Pittsburgh Epidemiology of Diabetes Complications study, a historical, prospective cohort study involving more than 600 type 1 diabetic individuals, demonstrated that insulin resistance (as measured by estimated glucose disposal rate) was predictive of hard cardiovascular outcomes, including death, nonfatal myocardial infarction, silent myocardial infarction, and significant coronary artery stenosis.[87] The obesity epidemic is likely more harmful in populations that are prone to developing diabetes, underscoring the genetic underpinnings of the problem. This point is supported by data from Italy showing that in this low-diabetes-risk population, only 0.2% of obese children were found to have type 2 diabetes.[88] This contrasts with the findings from a study of Mexican American youth living in south Texas, in which 82% of children with type 2 diabetes had a BMI greater than 25 kg/m^2.[89]

In addition to their obesity, children with type 2 diabetes often have other significant risk factors for cardiovascular disease, including high blood pressure and hyperlipidemia.[85] Although long-term data are limited in these individuals, one can theorize that a diagnosis of diabetes during childhood will lead to diabetes complications at an earlier age, and these may include heart, cerebrovascular, and renal diseases, among many others.[84] One study involving diabetic children in Australia found that type 2 diabetic children had higher rates of developing both hypertension and microalbuminuria than those of their peers with type 1 diabetes. Diabetic retinopathy, however, was more common in type 1 diabetic children.[90] In another study of 26 children with type 2 diabetes living in New York City, diabetic children were found to have significantly higher triglyceride concentrations and average systolic blood pressures, and 40% had microalbuminuria (with a mean duration of diabetes of 17 months).[91] These risk factors for the complications of diabetes can become quite expensive to treat and will likely be difficult for those from lower socioeconomic backgrounds to manage appropriately for this reason.

Diabetes in Minority Populations

Children and adolescents from minority populations, who are often living in lower-SES regions of the country and may have fewer resources available to them, are at particularly high risk for developing type 2 diabetes. One study of newly diagnosed, insulin-dependent diabetic individuals younger than 20 years in Allegheny County, Pennsylvania, found that in older adolescents (aged 15–19 years), the incidence of developing diabetes was almost 3 times higher in non-whites (30.4/100,000 people) than that in in whites (11.2/100,000).[92] This was a statistically significant difference (P = .001). Notably, this study did not differentiate between children with type 1 or type 2 diabetes. The authors noted that this was the first time in the history of their registry (which began recording patient information in 1965) that non-white children had a higher incidence of diabetes than did white children. They theorized that this increase in diabetes, particularly in adolescents aged 15 to 19 years, could be related to an increase in forms of diabetes besides "classical," insulin-dependent diabetes and suggested that this increase might be related to environmental changes, such as childhood weight gain.[92]

Other studies have supported the finding that the increase in type 2 diabetes in minority populations appears to increase with age. The previously described study of children living in south Texas from 1990 to 1998 found that 30% of Mexican American children had type 2 diabetes but that they accounted for 82% of the type 2 diabetes in children in that population.[89] The SEARCH for Diabetes in Youth study found that most children younger than 10 years of age with diabetes had type 1 disease.[8] Non-Hispanic white children made up the majority of these individuals (approximately 75%). However, children in this age group from minority populations (including African Americans, Hispanics, Asian/Pacific Islanders, and American Indians) were also more likely to have type 1 rather than type 2 diabetes. In children and adolescents aged 10 and older, however, the numbers were quite different. In these individuals, the majority were from minority populations (74%). Non-Hispanic whites continued to have a predominance of type 1 diabetes (85% of all cases). However, 58% of African American diabetics had type 2 disease, and in Asian/Pacific Islanders, the percentage was even higher at 70%. In American Indians with diabetes, a striking 86% of individuals had type 2 disease. Interestingly, Hispanic children in this age group still have more type 1 diabetes than type 2 (54% versus 46%) (**Table 6**).

Socioeconomics and the Increased Risk for Developing Diabetes

Lower SES is associated with an increased risk for developing diabetes. A subanalysis of data from NHANES III demonstrated that a lower SES (as defined by low income) was associated with a significantly increased risk for having type 2 diabetes in both African American and non-Hispanic white women.[93] Education level and occupation status were also associated with having diabetes in white women. Interestingly, there were no significant associations between SES and the risk for having type 2 diabetes in African American men. White men, however, were at increased risk as their income level decreased. Nelson and colleagues[94] found that children living in a mixed-race, urban (low-SES, high-poverty population), or rural working-class environment (low-SES, moderate-to-low minority population) were more likely to be overweight when compared with their peers living in newer suburban locations (high-SES, low-minority population). Another study of individuals in Alameda County, California, found that children who grew up with a lower socioeconomic position (as defined by the participant's father's occupation or education level) were more likely to develop type 2 diabetes.[95] As identified from the previous NHANES data, this finding was particularly

Table 6
Incidence rate of type 2 diabetes (reported with 95% confidence interval) in various age groups and ethnic populations

Incidence Rate of Type 2 Diabetes	
Age Group	Incidence Rate (With 95% Confidence Interval)
10–14 y	
Non-Hispanic white	3.0 (2.3–4.0)
African American	22.3 (18.1–27.5)
Hispanic	8.9 (6.4–12.3)
Asian/Pacific Islander	11.8 (7.9–17.5)
American Indian	25.3 (16.4–39.0)
15–19 y	
Non-Hispanic white	5.6 (4.5–6.9)
African American	19.4 (15.3–24.5)
Hispanic	17.0 (13.3–21.8)
Asian/Pacific Islander	22.7 (16.9–30.4)
American Indian	49.4 (35.6–68.5)

Data from Dabelea D, Bell RA, D'Agostino RB Jr., et al. Incidence of diabetes in youth in the United States. JAMA 2007;297(24):2716–24.

strong in women. The authors hypothesized that lower socioeconomic position was associated with risk factors for developing diabetes, including physical inactivity, limited opportunity for socioeconomic advancement, and poor nutrition.[95]

These socioeconomic differences do not carry over to the developing world, perhaps because of the relative scarcity of food resources in these countries. A study of schoolchildren living in Karachi, Pakistan, found that those living under low-income circumstances had fewer risk factors for developing diabetes than their middle-income counterparts. Children in middle-income groups were less active, watched more TV, were more likely to be overweight, and overall had a much stronger family history of diabetes.[96] This underscores the point that many of the factors behind increases in diabetes in the United States along socioeconomic lines may have much to do with the food and activity discrepancies seen in the developed world.

Socioeconomic Disparities in Caring for Diabetes

Diabetes is a very costly disease. According to a recent report from the American Diabetes Association (ADA), the total estimated cost from diabetes in the United States in 2007 was $174 billion dollars. Costs include both direct costs, such as visits to the doctor, hospitalizations related to diabetes complications and the costs of various pharmaceutical and blood glucose testing devices, as well as indirect costs, such as productivity time lost (estimated to be as much as $58 billion).[97] As much as 50% of these costs involve hospitalizations for inpatient care, and children and adolescents with diabetes are much less likely to incur these types of costs given their shorter duration of disease. However, as the number of children and adolescents with diabetes increases both in the United States and in countries around the world, one can project significantly higher future costs for all of these individuals, especially if they do not have access to proper preventive care and treatment. The ADA notes that medical costs for individuals with diabetes are more than twice that of someone without diabetes.[97] Although young children are not affected by loss of time at work, there are data from Canada suggesting that children with type 1 diabetes are more frequently absent from school.[98] One significant reason for absence was "poor meta-bolic control." Similar data for type 2 diabetes are not yet known.

Many individuals with chronic illnesses lack adequate health insurance, and those with diabetes are no exception. A recent study by Wilper and colleagues[99] found that almost 1.5 million working-age Americans with diabetes lacked health insurance and found that these individuals did not have the same access to health care as their insured counterparts. Further studies found that being uninsured was associated with having undetected diabetes, perhaps then increasing an individual's likelihood of developing preventable complications.[100] Some data regarding children and adoles-cents without adequate health insurance coverage also exist. In a study of type 1 dia-betic children and adolescents aged less than 20 years, underinsurance (patients without any health insurance, with Medicaid, or participating in their state's resident discount program) was associated with an increased risk of severe hypoglycemia. Older children without adequate insurance coverage had a relative risk of ketoacidosis that was more than 2 times that of those who had adequate insurance coverage.[101]

As the childhood and adolescent obesity epidemic continues to grow, so will the diabetes epidemic. We must develop better treatment and prevention strategies now if we are to stem this rising tide of disease and must focus much of our effort on caring for those minority and socioeconomic groups that are at highest risk.

TARGETED SOLUTIONS TO IMPROVING CHILDHOOD OBESITY AND DIABETES

The past decade has demonstrated that it will be difficult to decrease rates of child-hood obesity and diabetes, and it is also likely to be difficult to alter the societal patterns that result in socioeconomic discrepancies in obesity and diabetes. Improve-ments are likely to require large-scale interventions by government agencies and local communities. As one example, the obesity epidemic in the United States stimulated the 2001 US Surgeon General's *Call to Action to Prevent and Decrease Overweight and Obesity*, identifying 5 principles to guide the country toward a healthier lifestyle.[102] These principles included enhanced recognition of obesity as a health problem, as-sisting Americans in balancing their nutrition and exercise, identifying effective and culturally appropriate interventions, encouraging environmental changes to foster nutritious eating habits, and public-private partnerships to implement all of the above. Each decade, the government report "Healthy People" challenges individuals, communities and professionals to take specific steps to improve health. The most recent version, Healthy People 2010, not only outlined target percentages of adults and children who will be overweight or obese by 2010 but also directly addressed the inverse relationship of SES and childhood obesity among different races in Amer-ica.[103] The report identified obesity as a "result of a complex variety of social, behav-ioral, cultural, environmental, physiological and genetic factors." Due to the complexity of this issue, that report emphasized that initiatives designed to maintain a healthy weight should start in early childhood to increase the likelihood of healthy habits throughout adolescence and adulthood. The "Dietary Guidelines for Ameri-cans" is updated frequently and outlines nutritious guidelines for choosing food but has also started to address portion sizes in recent reports.[104]

Targeted Approaches to Improving Childhood Nutrition

For children, the US school system represents perhaps the most influential source of food away from home and a key area to target improvements. The opportunities for schools to positively impact the nutrition of US children have been limited by decreasing budgets, which have led to outsourcing food preparation and revenue-generating partnerships with manufacturers of energy-dense foods and beverages. The lost opportunity to provide abundant options for healthy food, rich in fruits and vegetables, to children from lower SES represents a great challenge to society. Although the prevalence of obesity in lower-SES families may be decreased only after decades of broad social reform, the protected school environment represents potential for rapid improvement in discrepancies in childhood food nutrition.

Some assistance has been offered by federal laws such as the 1994 "Healthy Meals for Healthy Americans Act" that required the NSBP and NSLP to meet the "Dietary Guidelines for Americans." In 2004, the "Child Nutrition and Nutrition Program for Women, Infants, and Children (WIC) Reauthorization Act" required school districts participating in the NSBP and NSLP to create "wellness" policies to include nutrition by the school year 2006 to 2007.[106] Further addressing the school environment, efforts such as the 2007 "Child Nutrition Promotion & School Lunch Protection Act" is seeking to change the definition of "food of minimal nutritional value" to reflect modern nutritional recommendations and broaden the power of the USDA to regulate all foods and beverages (vending machines, snack bars, etc.) sold in schools, not just food from federal school lunches.[106]

On a state level, collaborative alliances between the public and private sector have produced initiatives such as the 2006 "Alliance For A Healthier Generation—School Beverage Guidelines." The "Alliance for a Healthier Generation" is a joint initiative between the American Heart Association, the Clinton Foundation, and a number of food, beverage, and dairy companies designed to phase out full-calorie carbonated soft drinks and restrict snacks sold outside of the NSBP, with a goal of 100% compliance nationally by 2010. The strategy is to replace those goods with bottled water, low-fat and nonfat milk, 100% fruit juices, and low-calorie snacks. A 2008 progress report showed a 58% reduction of beverage calories shipped to US elementary, middle, and high schools under contract with such companies since 2004.

On a local level, school districts have the power to enact their own initiatives to further improve the nutritional environment of school children. In 2005, 25 schools in Mississippi combined distribution of free fruit and vegetables with nutrition-education activities for school children to increase consumption of healthier foods. Consumption of fruits inside school and overall increased significantly ($P=<0.01$) among eighth- and tenth-grade students; however, vegetable consumption inside school decreased significantly ($P=.05$) and remained unchanged overall.[107] A 1995 study of fourth- and fifth-grade students in a multiethnic school district in Minnesota combined behavioral curricula, parental involvement, school food-service changes, and industry support to promote fruit and vegetable consumption. The initiative increased lunchtime combined fruit and vegetable consumption, vegetable consumption in girls, as well as proportion of total daily calories from fruits and vegetables.[108] Individual school districts have taken the initiative to ban unhealthy snacks and carbonated soda sales to all school campuses. In 2004, the school board of the country's second largest school district, Los Angeles County, voted unanimously to ban unhealthy snacks and sugary carbonated beverages from its campuses.

The economic disparities in childhood and adult obesity are also being addressed at a local level through initiatives designed to alter the environment of poorer communities. Access to healthier options of affordable food is limited in low-income neighborhoods, making nearby fast food and full-service restaurant options more frequent choices for low-income families.[109] For this reason, a 2008 Los Angeles City Council ordinance was passed that prohibited construction of new fast-food restaurants in a 32 square-mile area of South Los Angeles, inhabited by 700,000 low-income people.

The goals of this ordinance were to allow city planners time to study the economic and environmental effects of overproliferation of fast-food restaurants in the community and develop solutions such as attracting full-service grocery stores, health food alternatives, and full-service restaurants.

Targeted Approaches to Increasing Childhood Activity

If we are going to make a difference in the obesity and diabetes epidemics affecting our children and adolescents, we must increase their physical activity and decrease their sedentary behaviors. More importantly, we must help them realize the importance of such lifestyle changes in improving their overall health. Various methods have been used to reach children to discuss these issues, and many of these have included children from lower socioeconomic backgrounds.

Marcus and colleagues reviewed and discussed many different media campaigns for improving physical activity. These included print and TV advertising, as well as radio announcements and mailings.[110] Unfortunately, although many of these programs improved awareness of the need to increase physical activity in a community, they did not necessarily increase activity. However, there have been successful interventions. The Physical Activity for Risk Reduction project involved a low-income community in Birmingham, Alabama, and hoped to improve and promote physical activity among its members. The intervention involved implementing various community programs and incorporated educational pamphlets. Although there were no statistically significant differences in activity levels between those in the intervention and those in the control groups at the study's completion, the study did show significant improvements in physical activity levels in areas of the community with stronger leadership and community organization.[110,111] This study suggested that in order for a campaign to be effective in promoting physical activity within a community, it must involve the leadership and existing organizational structure of that community.

Attempts to increase or improve physical activity during physical education in schools have also been evaluated. In France, a 4-year study of middle school students (Intervention Centered on Adolescents' Physical Activity and Sedentary Behavior) has been implemented, with goals of improving physical activity and education using the school as a central focus.[112] In this study, individuals participate in educational opportunities highlighting the importance of physical activity for one's health and also have increased opportunities both during and after school for increased physical activity and sports participation. Early, 6-month results indicate that participants are more involved in after-school physical activities (such as sports) and that students are involved in fewer sedentary behaviors (such as TV watching). Similar school-based programs have been completed or are underway in the United States, many of which have been reviewed by Stone and colleagues.[113] One, the Child and Adolescent Trial for Cardiovascular Health, studied elementary school-age children in 4 states, from various ethnic backgrounds.[114] They incorporated programs into the school curricula that promoted the importance of physical activity and in which increased physical activity is performed during physical education class. The program was able to increase the amount of moderate-to-vigorous physical activity among participants during the 3 years of the study. Importantly, follow-up studies of this group have indicated maintenance of these improved levels of physical activity for up to 3 years after the end of the official study period.[113]

These programs show that attitudes can change and physical activity levels can increase in child populations. We must be sure to target those at highest risk for decreased levels of physical activity and increased sedentary behavior, including those from lower socioeconomic backgrounds, and must direct our interventions to involve local community leadership and existing organizational structures. National, state, and local agencies must become involved in creating policies that will improve the physical activity and physical education of children. Along these lines, the US Congress has passed legislation such as the "Promoting Lifelong Active Communities Every Day Act," which promotes funding to help children, families, and communities achieve the national recommendation of 60 minutes of physical activity every day.[115] On the local level, the Florida Senate passed a bill setting clear guidelines for elementary school districts to comply with 150 min/wk of physical education. However, a major emphasis for prolonged change is likely to require parents to be involved to continue these improvements in activity at home.

Targeted Solution to Improving the Prevention and Care of Diabetes in Children

In order to reverse, or at the very least slow, the opidemic of type 2 diabetes in our children and adolescents, we must focus on programs that will improve the prevention of, screening for, and therapies for the disease. We cannot ignore those from lower socioeconomic and less-privileged backgrounds when producing and funding such interventions. Important programs are already in place, or are in development, and come from national, state, and community initiatives.

Lifestyle interventions, such as weight reduction, dietary changes, and increases in physical activity, have been shown to reduce the incidence of type 2 diabetes in adults at high risk for developing the disease.[116,117] Studies in children and adolescents are fewer, though some have been performed. These studies, such as the Kahnawake Schools Diabetes Prevention Project (involving school-age children in a Native American community near Montreal, Canada), the Bienestar Health Program (involving fourth-grade Mexican American children), and the Zuni Diabetes Prevention Program (targeting a Native American high school–age population),[118–121] demonstrate that community-based health education programs can have an impact on traditional risk factors for the development of type 2 diabetes. These include poor diet (high fat, low fruit and vegetable content) and increased sedentary behaviors (with associated paucity of more active behaviors).[118–120] However, 8-year follow-up results from the Kahnawake study demonstrated that improvements early during an intervention often do not persist and show the significant challenges confronted when attempting to alter a community's high-risk lifestyle behaviors.[121]

Any prevention program involving a large group of individuals will likely be expensive. This fact needs to be taken into consideration when developing such a program for any community, but particularly for a community with limited resources. In addition, the aforementioned studies have presented data regarding impacts on risk factors for the development of type 2 diabetes. Few data exist specifically addressing changes in the incidence of diabetes in a school-age population after such interventions. However, some studies have suggested a decrease in the prevalence of hyperinsulinemia, perhaps a surrogate for a prediabetic state.[119]

Early treatment of hyperglycemia and high blood pressure in type 2 diabetes has been shown to significantly reduce morbidity and mortality in adults.[122,123] This would indicate that earlier detection and treatment of diabetes should improve multiple outcomes, including the incidence of both micro- and macrovascular disease. Few data evaluating these clinical treatment outcomes in children with type 2 diabetes are available, making recommendations regarding screening less evidence based. However, the ADA recommends screening any child that is overweight or has at least 2 risk factors placing him or her at increased risk for having type 2 diabetes (including evidence of insulin resistance on clinical examination, such as acanthosis nigricans, hypertension, or hyperlipidemia; family history of diabetes; and particular ethnic background, such as Native American or African American). Fasting blood glucose values and oral glucose tolerance tests are considered appropriate screening methods.[124]

Importantly, not all children have equal access to the medical care necessary for the screening, diagnosis, and treatment of type 2 diabetes. Between 2000 and 2003, approximately 28% of US children lacked health insurance for at least some portion of the year.[125,126] Programs such as Medicaid and the Children's Health Insurance Program have been established to help overcome this critical hurdle to appropriate and necessary health care for children.[127] Studies have suggested that improved access to health care through such programs reduces emergency room visits, improves regular physician visits, and reduces family stress when children are provided proper coverage.[128] State and national governmental agencies must continue to do all that they can to ensure insurance coverage to as many children as possible, with a goal of improving preventive health care as well as improving the care of those already diagnosed with chronic diseases such as diabetes.

SUMMARY

In conclusion, the epidemic of obesity among children in the United States is due to multiple factors but is rooted in changes in food intake and physical activity among American children. Many factors related to both nutrition and activity have disproportionately affected children of lower SES. As our society attempts to act toward improving trends in pediatric obesity and diabetes, particular efforts should be made toward directing resources such that lower socioeconomic groups may benefit as well.

REFERENCES

1. Ogden CL, Carroll MD, Flegal KM. High body mass index for age among US children and adolescents, 2003–2006. JAMA 2008;299(20):2401–5.
2. Freedman DS, Dietz WH, Srinivasan SR, et al. The relation of overweight to cardiovascular risk factors among children and adolescents: the Bogalusa Heart Study. Pediatrics 1999;103(6 Pt 1):1175–82.
3. Webber LS, Osganian V, Luepker RV, et al. Cardiovascular risk factors among third grade children in four regions of the United States. The CATCH Study. Child and adolescent trial for cardiovascular health. Am J Epidemiol 1995;141(5): 428–39.
4. McNiece KL, Poffenbarger TS, Turner JL, et al. Prevalence of hypertension and pre-hypertension among adolescents. J Pediatr 2007;150(6):640–4, 644.e1.
5. Sorof JM, Turner J, Franco K, et al. Characteristics of hypertensive children identified by primary care referral compared with school-based screening. J Pediatr 2004;144(4):485–9.
6. Sinha R, Fisch G, Teague B, et al. Prevalence of impaired glucose tolerance among children and adolescents with marked obesity. N Engl J Med 2002; 346(11):802–10.
7. Weiss R, Dziura J, Burgert TS, et al. Obesity and the metabolic syndrome in children and adolescents. N Engl J Med 2004;350(23):2362–74.
8. Dabelea D, Bell RA, D'Agostino RB Jr, et al. Incidence of diabetes in youth in the United States. JAMA 2007;297(24):2716–24.
9. Franks PW, Hanson RL, Knowler WC, et al. Childhood predictors of young-onset type 2 diabetes. Diabetes 2007;56(12):2964–72.

10. Strauss RS, Barlow SE, Dietz WH. Prevalence of abnormal serum aminotransferase values in overweight and obese adolescents. J Pediatr 2000;136(6):727–33.
11. Narayan KM, Boyle JP, Thompson TJ, et al. Lifetime risk for diabetes mellitus in the United States. JAMA 2003;290(14):1884–90.
12. Delva J, Johnston LD, O'Malley PM. The epidemiology of overweight and related lifestyle behaviors: racial/ethnic and socioeconomic status differences among American youth. Am J Prev Med 2007;33(4 Suppl):S178–86.
13. Kumanyika S, Grier S. Targeting interventions for ethnic minority and low-income populations. Future Child 2006;16(1):187–207.
14. Rolls BJ, Drewnowski A, Ledikwe JH. Changing the energy density of the diet as a strategy for weight management. J Am Diet Assoc 2005;105(5 Suppl 1):S98–103.
15. Ledikwe JH, Ello-Martin JA, Rolls BJ. Portion sizes and the obesity epidemic. J Nutr 2005;135(4):905–9.
16. McCrory MA, Fuss PJ, McCallum JE, et al. Dietary variety within food groups: association with energy intake and body fatness in men and women. Am J Clin Nutr 1999;69(3):440–7.
17. Rolls BJ, Roe LS, Meengs JS. The effect of large portion sizes on energy intake is sustained for 11 days. Obesity (Silver Spring) 2007;15(6):1535–43.
18. Nestle M, Jacobson MF. Halting the obesity epidemic: a public health policy approach. Public Health Rep 2000;115(1):12–24.
19. Freedman DS, Khan LK, Serdula MK, et al. Racial and ethnic differences in secular trends for childhood BMI, weight, and height. Obesity (Silver Spring) 2006;14(2):301–8.
20. Kilmer G, Roberts H, Hughes E, et al. Surveillance of certain health behaviors and conditions among states and selected local areas–Behavioral Risk Factor Surveillance System (BRFSS), United States, 2006. MMWR Surveill Summ 2008;57(7):1–188.
21. Powell LM, Slater S, Mirtcheva D, et al. Food store availability and neighborhood characteristics in the United States. Prev Med 2007;44(3):189–95.
22. Glanz K, Sallis JF, Saelens BE, et al. Nutrition Environment Measures Survey in stores (NEMS-S): development and evaluation. Am J Prev Med 2007;32(4):282–9.
23. Ogden CL, Carroll MD, Curtin LR, et al. Prevalence of overweight and obesity in the United States, 1999–2004. JAMA 2006;295(13):1549–55.
24. Chang VW, Lauderdale DS. Income disparities in body mass index and obesity in the United States, 1971–2002. Arch Intern Med 2005;165(18):2122–8.
25. Paeratakul S, Lovejoy JC, Ryan DH, et al. The relation of gender, race and socioeconomic status to obesity and obesity comorbidities in a sample of US adults. Int J Obes Relat Metab Disord 2002;26(9):1205–10.
26. Freedman DS, Ogden CL, Flegal KM, et al. Childhood overweight and family income. MedGenMed 2007;9(2):26.
27. Cohany SR, Emy S. Trends of labor force participation of married mothers of infants. Mon Labor Rev 2007;130(2):9–16.
28. Nestle M. Food politics- how the food industry influences nutrition and health. Berkeley (CA): University of California Press; 2007.
29. McNeal J. Marketing to kids: myths and realities. Ithaca (NY): Paramount Market Publishing, Inc; 1999.
30. Cavadini C, Siega-Riz AM, Popkin BM. US adolescent food intake trends from 1965 to 1996. Arch Dis Child 2000;83(1):18–24.

31. Powell LM, Szczypka G, Chaloupka FJ. Adolescent exposure to food advertising on television. Am J Prev Med 2007;33(4 Suppl):S251–6.
32. Bhattacharya J, DeLeire T, Haider S, et al. Heat or eat? Cold-weather shocks and nutrition in poor American families. Am J Public Health 2003;93(7):1149–54.
33. Chao EL, Utgoff KP. 100 Years of U.S. Consumer Spending; Data for the Nation, New York City, and Boston. May 2006, U.S. Department of Labor Report 991.
34. Lin BH, Guthrie J, Frazao E. Away-from-home foods increasingly important to quality of American diet. Economic Research Service, USDA, FDA, DHHS Agriculture Information, Bulletin No. 749. Washington DC, 1999.
35. Nielsen SJ, Siega-Riz AM, Popkin BM. Trends in energy intake in U.S. between 1977 and 1996: similar shifts seen across age groups. Obes Res 2002;10(5):370–8.
36. United_States_Department-of_Agriculture. Nutrition program facts. Alexandria (VA): United States Department of Agriculture; 2002.
37. Wang Y. Cross-national comparison of childhood obesity: the epidemic and the relationship between obesity and socioeconomic status. Int J Epidemiol 2001;30(5):1129–36.
38. Critser G. Fat land. New York: Houghton Mifflin Company; 2003.
39. United_States_Department-of_Agriculture. USDA school nutrition dietary assessment study-III. Alexandria (VA): United States Department of Agriculture; 1997.
40. Johnston LD, Delva J, O'Malley PM. Soft drink availability, contracts, and revenues in American secondary schools. Am J Prev Med 2007;33(4 Suppl):S209–25.
41. Guthrie JF, Morton JF. Food sources of added sweeteners in the diets of Americans. J Am Diet Assoc 2000;100(1):43–51, quiz 49–50.
42. Ballew C, Kuester S, Gillespie C. Beverage choices affect adequacy of children's nutrient intakes. Arch Pediatr Adolesc Med 2000;154(11):1148–52.
43. Marshall TA, Eichenberger Gilmore JM, Broffitt B, et al. Diet quality in young children is influenced by beverage consumption. J Am Coll Nutr 2005;24(1):65–75.
44. Ludwig DS, Peterson KE, Gortmaker SL. Relation between consumption of sugar-sweetened drinks and childhood obesity: a prospective, observational analysis. Lancet 2001;357(9255):505–8.
45. O'Malley PM, Johnston LD, Delva J, et al. Variation in obesity among American secondary school students by school and school characteristics. Am J Prev Med 2007;33(4 Suppl):S187–94.
46. Slusser WM, Cumberland WG, Browdy BL, et al. Overweight in urban, low-income, African American and Hispanic children attending Los Angeles elementary schools: research stimulating action. Public Health Nutr 2005;8(2):141–8.
47. Dencker M, Andersen LB. Health-related aspects of objectively measured daily physical activity in children. Clin Physiol Funct Imaging 2008;28(3):133–44.
48. Corder K, Ekelund U, Steele RM, et al. Assessment of physical activity in youth. J Appl Phys 2008;105(3):977–87.
49. Rowlands AV. Accelerometer assessment of physical activity in children: an update. Pediatr Exerc Sci 2007;19(3):252–66.
50. Daniels SR, Arnett DK, Eckel RH, et al. Overweight in children and adolescents: pathophysiology, consequences, prevention, and treatment. Circulation 2005;111(15):1999–2012.
51. Nader PR, Bradley RH, Houts RM, et al. Moderate-to-vigorous physical activity from ages 9 to 15 years. JAMA 2008;300(3):295–305.
52. Troiano RP, Berrigan D, Dodd KW, et al. Physical activity in the United States measured by accelerometer. Med Sci Sports Exerc 2008;40(1):181–8.

53. Eisenmann JC, Bartee RT, Wang MQ. Physical activity, TV viewing, and weight in U.S. youth: 1999 youth risk behavior survey. Obes Res 2002;10(5):379–85.
54. Guo SS, Roche AF, Chumlea WC, et al. The predictive value of childhood body mass index values for overweight at age 35 y. Am J Clin Nutr 1994; 59(4):810–9.
55. Pinhas-Hamiel O, Dolan LM, Daniels SR, et al. Increased incidence of non-insulin-dependent diabetes mellitus among adolescents. J Pediatr 1996;128(5 Pt 1):608–15.
56. Grinstein G, Muzumdar R, Aponte L, et al. Presentation and 5-year follow-up of type 2 diabetes mellitus in African-American and Caribbean-Hispanic adolescents. Horm Res 2003;60(3):121–6.
57. Hu FB, Leitzmann MF, Stampfer MJ, et al. Physical activity and television watching in relation to risk for type 2 diabetes mellitus in men. Arch Intern Med 2001; 161(12):1542–8.
58. Hu FB, Li TY, Colditz GA, et al. Television watching and other sedentary behaviors in relation to risk of obesity and type 2 diabetes mellitus in women. JAMA 2003;289(14):1785–91.
59. Margeirsdottir HD, Larsen JR, Brunborg C, et al. Strong association between time watching television and blood glucose control in children and adolescents with type 1 diabetes. Diabetes Care 2007;30(6):1567–70.
60. Strauss RS, Rodzilsky D, Burack G, et al. Psychosocial correlates of physical activity in healthy children. Arch Pediatr Adolesc Med 2001;155(8):897–902.
61. Wang F, Veugelers PJ. Self-esteem and cognitive development in the era of the childhood obesity epidemic. Obes Rev 2008;9(6):615–23.
62. Kemper HC, Twisk JW, van Mechelen W, et al. A fifteen-year longitudinal study in young adults on the relation of physical activity and fitness with the development of the bone mass: The Amsterdam Growth And Health Longitudinal Study. Bone 2000;27(6):847–53.
63. Bakker I, Twisk JW, Van Mechelen W, et al. Ten-year longitudinal relationship between physical activity and lumbar bone mass in (young) adults. J Bone Miner Res 2003;18(2):325–32.
64. Pate RR, Heath GW, Dowda M, et al. Associations between physical activity and other health behaviors in a representative sample of US adolescents. Am J Public Health 1996;86(11):1577–81.
65. Pivarnik JM, Bray MS, Hergenroeder AC, et al. Ethnicity affects aerobic fitness in US adolescent girls. Med Sci Sports Exerc 1995;27(12):1635–8.
66. Simons-Morton BG, McKenzie TJ, Stone E, et al. Physical activity in a multi-ethnic population of third graders in four states. Am J Public Health 1997; 87(1):45–50.
67. Lindquist CH, Reynolds KD, Goran MI. Sociocultural determinants of physical activity among children. Prev Med 1999;29(4):305–12.
68. Johnston LD, Delva J, O'Malley PM. Sports participation and physical education in American secondary schools: current levels and racial/ethnic and socioeconomic disparities. Am J Prev Med 2007;33(4 Suppl):S195–208.
69. Andersen RE, Crespo CJ, Bartlett SJ, et al. Relationship of physical activity and television watching with body weight and level of fatness among children: results from the third national health and nutrition examination survey. JAMA 1998; 279(12):938–42.
70. Brodersen NH, Steptoe A, Boniface DR, et al. Trends in physical activity and sedentary behaviour in adolescence: ethnic and socioeconomic differences. Br J Sports Med 2007;41(3):140–4.

71. Graves L, Stratton G, Ridgers ND, et al. Comparison of energy expenditure in adolescents when playing new generation and sedentary computer games: cross sectional study. BMJ 2007;335(7633):1282–4.
72. Gordon-Larsen P, Nelson MC, Page P, et al. Inequality in the built environment underlies key health disparities in physical activity and obesity. Pediatrics 2006;117(2):417–24.
73. From the Centers for Disease Control and Prevention. Adult blood lead epidemiology and surveillance. JAMA 1993;269(11):1373.
74. Loukaitou-Sideris A, Eck JE. Crime prevention and active living. Am J Health Promot 2007;21(4 Suppl):380–9, iii.
75. Burdette HL, Whitaker RC. A national study of neighborhood safety, outdoor play, television viewing, and obesity in preschool children. Pediatrics 2005; 116(3):657–62.
76. Romero AJ, Robinson TN, Kraemer HC, et al. Are perceived neighborhood hazards a barrier to physical activity in children? Arch Pediatr Adolesc Med 2001;155(10):1143–8.
77. Anderssen N, Wold B. Parental and peer influences on leisure-time physical activity in young adolescents. Res Q Exerc Sport 1992;63(4):341–8.
78. Cowie CC, Rust KF, Byrd-Holt DD, et al. Prevalence of diabetes and impaired fasting glucose in adults in the U.S. population: National Health And Nutrition Examination Survey 1999–2002. Diabetes Care 2006;29(6):1263–8.
79. CDC. "Diabetes Fact Sheet 2007". Available at: http://www.cdc.gov/diabetes/pubs/pdf/ndfs_2007.pdf. Accessed December 1, 2008.
80. Wild S, Roglic G, Green A, et al. Global prevalence of diabetes: estimates for the year 2000 and projections for 2030. Diabetes Care 2004;27(5):1047–53.
81. Rosenbloom AL, Joe JR, Young RS, et al. Emerging epidemic of type 2 diabetes in youth. Diabetes Care 1999;22(2):345–54.
82. Connolly V, Unwin N, Sherriff P, et al. Diabetes prevalence and socioeconomic status: a population based study showing increased prevalence of type 2 diabetes mellitus in deprived areas. J Epidemiol Community Health 2000;54(3): 173–7.
83. Type 2 diabetes in children and adolescents. American Diabetes Association. Diabetes Care 2000;23(3):381–9.
84. Fagot-Campagna A, Pettitt DJ, Engelgau MM, et al. Type 2 diabetes among North American children and adolescents: an epidemiologic review and a public health perspective. J Pediatr 2000;136(5):664–72.
85. Steinberger J, Daniels SR. Obesity, insulin resistance, diabetes, and cardiovascular risk in children: an American Heart Association scientific statement from the Atherosclerosis, Hypertension, and Obesity in the young committee (Council on Cardiovascular Disease in the Young) and the diabetes committee (Council on Nutrition, Physical Activity, and Metabolism). Circulation 2003;107(10): 1448–53.
86. Williams KV, Erbey JR, Becker D, et al. Can clinical factors estimate insulin resistance in type 1 diabetes? Diabetes 2000;49(4):626–32.
87. Orchard TJ, Olson JC, Erbey JR, et al. Insulin resistance-related factors, but not glycemia, predict coronary artery disease in type 1 diabetes: 10-year follow-up data from the Pittsburgh epidemiology of diabetes complications study. Diabetes Care 2003;26(5):1374–9.
88. Invitti C, Guzzaloni G, Gilardini L, et al. Prevalence and concomitants of glucose intolerance in European obese children and adolescents. Diabetes Care 2003; 26(1):118–24.

89. Hale DE, Rupert G. The changing spectrum of diabetes in Mexican American youth. Rev Endocr Metab Disord 2006;7(3):163–70.

90. Eppens MC, Craig ME, Cusumano J, et al. Prevalence of diabetes complications in adolescents with type 2 compared with type 1 diabetes. Diabetes Care 2006; 29(6):1300–6.

91. Ettinger LM, Freeman K, DiMartino-Nardi JR, et al. Microalbuminuria and abnormal ambulatory blood pressure in adolescents with type 2 diabetes mellitus. J Pediatr 2005;147(1):67–73.

92. Libman IM, LaPorte RE, Becker D, et al. Was there an epidemic of diabetes in nonwhite adolescents in Allegheny County, Pennsylvania? Diabetes Care 1998;21(8):1278–81.

93. Robbins JM, Vaccarino V, Zhang H, et al. Socioeconomic status and type 2 diabetes in African American and non Hicpanic white women and men: evidence from the third national health and nutrition examination survey. Am J Public Health 2001;91(1):76–83.

94. Nelson MC, Gordon-Larsen P, Song Y, et al. Built and social environments: associations with adolescent overweight and activity. Am J Prev Med 2006;31(2):109–17.

95. Maty SC, Lynch JW, Raghunathan TE, et al. Childhood socioeconomic position, gender, adult body mass index, and incidence of type 2 diabetes mellitus over 34 years in the Alameda County Study. Am J Public Health 2008;98(8):1486–94.

96. Hydrie MZ, Basit A, Ahmedani MY, et al. Comparison of risk factors for diabetes in children of different socioeconomic status. J Coll Physicians Surg Pak 2005; 15(2):74–7.

97. American Diabetes Association. Economic costs of diabetes in the U.S. in 2007. Diabetes Care 2008;31(3):596–615.

98. Glaab LA, Brown R, Daneman D. School attendance in children with type 1 diabetes. Diabet Med 2005;22(4):421–6.

99. Wilper AP, Woolhandler S, Lasser KE, et al. A national study of chronic disease prevalence and access to care in uninsured U.S. adults. Ann Intern Med 2008; 149(3):170–6.

100. Zhang X, Geiss LS, Cheng YJ, et al. The missed patient with diabetes: how access to health care affects the detection of diabetes. Diabetes Care 2008; 31(9):1748–53.

101. Rewers A, Chase HP, Mackenzie T, et al. Predictors of acute complications in children with type 1 diabetes. JAMA 2002;287(19):2511–8.

102. U.S. Department of Health and Human Services. The Surgeon General's Call to Action to Prevent and Decrease Overweight and Obesity; 2001.

103. US Department of Health and Human Services. Healthy people 2010: understanding and improving health. 2nd edition. Washington, DC: US Government Printing Office; 2000.

104. US Department of Health and Human Services and US Department of Agriculture. Dietary guidelines for Americans, 2005. 6th edition. Washington, D.C.: US Government Printing Office; 2005.

105. Masse LC, Frosh MM, Chriqui JF, et al. Development of a School Nutrition-Environment State Policy Classification System (SNESPCS). Am J Prev Med 2007; 33(4 Suppl):S277–91.

106. GovTrack.us. S. 771–110th Congress (2007): Child Nutrition Promotion and School Lunch Protection Act of 2007. Available at: http://www.govtrack.us/congress/bill.xpd?bill=h110-1363&tab=related. Accessed March 18, 2009.

107. CDC. Evaluation of a fruit and vegetable distribution program—Mississippi, 2004–05 School Year. MMWR Morb Mortal Wkly Rep 2006;55(35):957–61.

108. Perry CL, Bishop DB, Taylor G, et al. Changing fruit and vegetable consumption among children: the 5-a-day power plus program in St. Paul, Minnesota. Am J Public Health 1998;88(4):603–9.
109. Ayala GX, Mueller K, Lopez-Madurga E, et al. Restaurant and food shopping selections among Latino women in Southern California. J Am Diet Assoc 2005;105(1):38–45.
110. Marcus BH, Owen N, Forsyth LH, et al. Physical activity interventions using mass media, print media, and information technology. Am J Prev Med 1998; 15(4):362–78.
111. Lewis CE, Raczynski JM, Heath GW Jr, et al. Promoting physical activity in low-income African-American communities: the PARR project. Ethn Dis 1993;3(2): 106–18.
112. Simon C, Wagner A, Platat C, et al. ICAPS: a multilevel program to improve physical activity in adolescents. Diabetes Metab 2006;32(1):41–9.
113. Stone EJ, McKenzie TL, Welk GJ, et al. Effects of physical activity interventions in youth. Review and synthesis. Am J Prev Med 1998;15(4):298–315.
114. Luepker RV, Perry CL, McKinlay SM, et al. Outcomes of a field trial to improve children's dietary patterns and physical activity. The child and adolescent trial for cardiovascular health. CATCH collaborative group. JAMA 1996;275(10): 768–76.
115. GovTrack.us. S. 1342–110th Congress (2007): Healthy Lifestyles and Prevention America Act; 2007. Available at: http://www.govtrack.us/congress/bill. xpd?bill=h110-2633. Accessed March 18, 2009.
116. Tuomilehto J, Lindstrom J, Eriksson JG, et al. Prevention of type 2 diabetes mellitus by changes in lifestyle among subjects with impaired glucose tolerance. N Engl J Med 2001;344(18):1343–50.
117. Knowler WC, Barrett-Connor E, Fowler SE, et al. Reduction in the incidence of type 2 diabetes with lifestyle intervention or metformin. N Engl J Med 2002; 346(6):393–403.
118. Macaulay AC, Paradis G, Potvin L, et al. The Kahnawake schools diabetes prevention project: intervention, evaluation, and baseline results of a diabetes primary prevention program with a native community in Canada. Prev Med 1997;26(6):779–90.
119. Teufel NI, Ritenbaugh CK. Development of a primary prevention program: insight gained in the Zuni diabetes prevention program. Clin Pediatr (Phila) 1998;37(2):131–41.
120. Trevino RP, Pugh JA, Hernandez AE, et al. Bienestar: a diabetes risk-factor prevention program. J Sch Health 1998;68(2):62–7.
121. Paradis G, Levesque L, Macaulay AC, et al. Impact of a diabetes prevention program on body size, physical activity, and diet among Kanien'keha:ka (Mohawk) children 6 to 11 years old: 8-year results from the Kahnawake Schools Diabetes Prevention Project. Pediatrics 2005;115(2):333–9.
122. Holman RR, Paul SK, Bethel MA, et al. 10-year follow-up of intensive glucose control in type 2 diabetes. N Engl J Med 2008;359(15):1577–89.
123. Holman RR, Paul SK, Bethel MA, et al. Long-term follow-up after tight control of blood pressure in type 2 diabetes. N Engl J Med 2008;359(15):1565–76.
124. Ludwig DS, Ebbeling CB. Type 2 diabetes mellitus in children: primary care and public health considerations. JAMA 2001;286(12):1427–30.
125. Olson LM, Tang SF, Newacheck PW. Children in the United States with discontinuous health insurance coverage. N Engl J Med 2005;353(4):382–91.

126. Cassedy A, Fairbrother G, Newacheck PW. The impact of insurance instability on children's access, utilization, and satisfaction with health care. Ambul Pediatr 2008;8(5):321–8.

127. Sommers BD. Protecting low-income children's access to care: are physician visits associated with reduced patient dropout from Medicaid and the children's health insurance program? Pediatrics 2006;118(1):e36–42.

128. Lave JR, Keane CR, Lin CJ, et al. Impact of a children's health insurance program on newly enrolled children. JAMA 1998;279(22):1820–5.

Pre-Exercise Cardiology Screening Guidelines for Asymptomatic Patients with Diabetes

Siddhartha S. Angadi, B.O.Th*, Glenn A. Gaesser, PhD

KEYWORDS

- Diabetes • Exercise • Screening
- Cardiovascular disease risk • Asymptomatic
- Silent myocardial ischemia

Coronary artery disease (CAD) is the leading cause of death in patients with diabetes mellitus. Studies have shown that patients with type 2 diabetes (T2D) are 2 to 5 times more likely to die from heart disease,[1] and CAD accounts for approximately 65% to 80% of deaths in diabetic patients.[2] A similar trend has been observed in patients with type 1 diabetes (T1D).[3–5] For example, data from the Pittsburgh insulin-dependent diabetes mellitus morbidity and mortality study reported a 10-fold greater CAD mortality compared with expected mortality rates from United States national data.[3]

Exercise is a cornerstone in the treatment and management of diabetes not only for improving glycemic control but also for reducing CAD morbidity and mortality. Cardiorespiratory fitness is inversely associated with morbidity and mortality in persons with diabetes.[6,7] Therefore, an important clinical goal should be to increase cardiorespiratory fitness of individuals with diabetes. Exercise is suitable for achieving this goal and thus is recommended for persons with diabetes.[8,9] However, to maximize benefit and minimize risk, pre-exercise evaluation should be considered. For patients with asymptomatic diabetes, the extent to which pre-exercise screening is necessary is controversial.[10,11] Routine CAD screening for CAD-asymptomatic patients with diabetes does not have strong evidence-based support.[12] However, it may be possible to use multiple screening tools to help identify those persons with diabetes for whom pre-exercise cardiology screening is warranted.

Although it is clear that CAD is a major problem in the diabetic population, screening for latent CAD is problematic because silent myocardial ischemia (SMI), or

Department of Exercise and Wellness, Arizona State University, 7350 E. Unity Avenue, Mesa, AZ 85296, USA
* Corresponding author.
E-mail address: siddhartha.angadi@asu.edu (S.S. Angadi).

Clin Sports Med 28 (2009) 379–392
doi:10.1016/j.csm.2009.02.002
0278-5919/09/$ – see front matter © 2009 Elsevier Inc. All rights reserved.

asymptomatic myocardial ischemia, is commonly present in patients with T1D and T2D. SMI is uniformly associated with poor outcomes in patients with T2D, with studies showing increased risk of cardiac events ranging from 3-fold[13] to 21-fold.[14] The prognostic implications of SMI in T1D have not been reported but it is probable that the risk profile would be similar, if not worse than in T2D.

The prevalence of SMI in populations with T2D ranges from 17% to 22% on functional cardiac testing (eg, exercise stress test, myocardial perfusion scan).[15,16] The incidence of SMI in T1D ranges from 11% to 34%.[17] As a result, diagnosis of CAD is delayed and these patients are more likely to have triple vessel or multiple vessel coronary artery disease along with derangements in systolic and diastolic function.[18,19]

The purpose of this review is to discuss the relevant issues regarding pre-exercise cardiology screening in asymptomatic patients with diabetes, and to present options with regard to guidelines for pre-exercise screening in this population.

EPIDEMIOLOGY OF SMI IN PATIENTS WITH T2D

Fornengo and colleagues[15] found that 17% of individuals with T2D who underwent a graded exercise test in the absence of traditional cardiovascular risk factors (eg, dyslipidemia, hypertension, peripheral vascular disease, retinopathy, microalbuminuria) and with a negative history of heart disease had a positive exercise stress test. Wackers and colleagues[16] noted in the Detection of Ischemia in Asymptomatic Diabetics (DIAD) study that 22% of persons with T2D, who underwent adenosine technetium-99 sestamibi single photon emission computed tomography (SPECT), had silent ischemia. Furthermore, moderate-to-large perfusion defects were observed in 40% of those who had an abnormal stress test.

In individuals with T1D, functional cardiac testing revealed an 11% incidence of SMI,[17] whereas imaging with either coronary angiography or a dual strategy of angiography plus intravascular ultrasound revealed incidence rates of 4.2 and 34%, respectively.[17,20] The large discrepancy between the 2 studies is plausible because Janand-Delenne and colleagues[17] used only coronary angiography, which is known to underestimate the true extent of CAD (compared with coronary angiography + intravascular ultrasound). In addition, only patients with positive exercise tests had angiography. However, angiographic disease severity is not a reliable predictor of myocardial ischemia.

POTENTIAL BENEFITS OF EARLY DIAGNOSIS OF SMI

Few studies have evaluated the changes in inducible ischemia over time in patients with T2D. A significant finding from the DIAD study revealed that 79% of patients who had perfusion abnormalities at the time of enrollment, had complete resolution of their perfusion defects at 3-year follow-up as a result of intensive medical treatment of their risk factors with aspirin, statins, and angiotensin converting enzyme inhibitors.[21] Ischemic perfusion abnormalities in this patient population seem to be primarily as a result of either or both microvascular and macrovascular endothelial dysfunction. Although the benefits of exercise in this population have yet to be tested, exercise has been shown to favorably modify this aspect of the disease process. Therefore, it is possible that a noninvasive strategy using drug therapy coupled with lifestyle modifications and exercise could have a positive impact in this population. Definitive outcome studies need to be performed.

Another therapeutic approach could be the adoption of an invasive revascularization strategy in these patients. A small open-label pilot study by Faglia and colleagues[22] demonstrated a 16% reduction in adverse events associated with

SMI. In a small study conducted at the Mayo Clinic, patients with high-risk SPECT scans appeared to have a survival advantage after undergoing coronary artery bypass graft compared with percutaneous coronary intervention or medical management.[23] However, there have been no large prospective studies to judge the true value of this therapeutic approach.

IS PRE-EXERCISE SCREENING NECESSARY?

Exercise is associated with a transient increase in the risk of sudden cardiac death.[24–26] Diabetes is also considered a risk factor for sudden unexpected cardiac death.[27] However, the risk is significantly reduced in patients who undergo habitual physical activity.[28] Therefore, pre-exercise screening could conceivably reduce the risk of a cardiac event in a diabetic patient before commencement of an exercise program. Aerobic exercise is a potent CAD risk modifier and an essential component of a diabetes management program since it enhances skeletal muscle insulin sensitivity. As a result of exercise training interventions, total and cardiovascular mortality in patients with a history of myocardial infarction is reduced by 27% and 31%, respectively.[29] Although its usefulness in resolving SMI remains untested, favorable results of exercise interventions in patients with occlusive CAD[30,31] suggest that exercise intervention programs could reduce morbidity and mortality in this population.

EVALUATION AND TESTING FOR SMI
Identifying Patients at Increased Risk for SMI

Predicting SMI is difficult. The American Diabetes Association (ADA) published guidelines in 1998 to facilitate the identification of patients at risk.[32] These guidelines recommended specialized CAD screening for patients considered to be high risk, and focused on the number, rather than the severity of CAD risk factors, in asymptomatic and symptomatic individuals.

These recommendations have since been challenged on the basis of results from several studies.[16,33,34] For example, in the DIAD study, most patients with SMI had few traditional and novel risk factors associated with CAD including hypertension, smoking, dyslipidemia, high-sensitivity C-reactive protein, homocysteine, lipid subfractions, and plasminogen activator inhibitor-1, which in turn were not predictive of an abnormal SPECT test.[16] These findings should, however, be tempered by the fact that tests used to detect SMI may not necessarily accurately identify patients at increased risk for either acute plaque rupture, thrombosis, myocardial infarction, or death.[12,35,36]

In T1D, strong predictors of SMI seem to be a family history of CAD, peripheral arterial disease, disease duration,[32] and microangiopathic changes including either retinopathy or nephropathy.[37] Diabetic retinopathy may also serve as a surrogate marker of SMI because it has been shown to be associated with a reduction in coronary flow reserve in patients with diabetes.[38]

Men seem to have a higher risk of silent ischemia.[16] Although the absolute risk of cardiovascular events is higher in men than in women, the relative risk is higher in women than in men.[39] Erectile dysfunction (ED) in men has also been implicated as a predictor of SMI because ED is most likely due to early stage atherosclerosis and endothelial dysfunction.[40] The risk factors for ED are similar to those of CAD and include smoking, hypertension, dyslipidemia, diabetes, and lack of physical activity. Notably, ED remains a risk factor for adverse cardiac events even after adjusting for these risk factors.[41,42]

Laboratory Tests

Two simple laboratory tests, microalbuminuria and glycosylated hemoglobin (HbA_{1c}), can help stratify the risk of SMI in patients with diabetes.

Microalbuminuria

SMI seems to be more common in patients with type 2 diabetes who have microalbuminuria, which is strongly predictive of an ischemic response to exercise testing[43] and tends to be associated with longer duration of diabetes and with impairment of endothelium-dependent flow-mediated dilation, a known risk factor for CAD.[44] Microalbuminuria also predicts the development of overt nephropathy in patients with diabetes. Chronic kidney disease in the setting of T2D carries a poor prognosis with 40% of patients experiencing a cardiac event over a 5-year period.[45] However, in the DIAD study, microalbuminuria was not predictive of an increased risk of inducible ischemia.[16]

Poor glycemic control

Because long-term glycemic control is a significant predictor of angiographically apparent coronary artery disease,[20] individuals with poor glycemic control may be at enhanced risk for SMI. However, the correlation between HbA_{1c} and SMI is controversial. Whereas some studies have shown an association between SMI and HbA_{1c}, with high HbA_{1c} values predictive of abnormal myocardial perfusion scans and stenotic segments on coronary angiography,[46] others have not.[17,43,47–49] HbA_{1c} seems to be more predictive of microvascular complications than macrovascular complications in patients with diabetes.[50,51] In a small study of patients with T1D, long-term glycemic control was found to be predictive of angiographically significant stenosis.[20]

Bedside Tests

Simple bedside tests for peripheral arterial disease, autonomic dysfunction, and a resting ECG, may also be of considerable value when screening for SMI.

Peripheral arterial disease

A thorough clinical history, as well as physical examination for bruits and peripheral pulses, is important for the detection of peripheral atherosclerotic disease. The ankle–brachial index is an easy-to-use bedside test for peripheral arterial disease and is also a specific indicator for the risk of future CAD events. A low ankle-brachial index has sensitivity of 16.5% and specificity of 92.7% to predict future CAD, and sensitivity of 41% and specificity of 88% to predict future cardiac death.[52] Approximately 5% of patients with peripheral arterial disease will have a falsely elevated ankle–brachial index (>0.9) due to arterial calcification.[53]

Autonomic neuropathy

The presence of autonomic neuropathy was found to be a strong predictor of an abnormal perfusion scan in the DIAD study.[16] Patients with an abnormal Valsalva response had a 5.6-fold increased risk of an abnormal SPECT study. In a small study of 12 diabetic patients, Baxter and colleagues[54] found that patients with SMI consistently had a worse autonomic score when they underwent 5 well-validated and standardized autonomic function tests. The tests of autonomic function used were:

1. R-R interval variation with respiration (parasympathetic)
2. R-R interval variation with the Valsalva maneuver (parasympathetic)
3. supine and erect blood pressure (sympathetic)
4. supine and erect heart rate (parasympathetic)
5. blood pressure response to sustained handgrip (sympathetic)

Each test was scored 0 (normal), 1 (borderline), or 2 (abnormal), and all 5 tests were then used to compile an autonomic score between 0 and 10. The SMI group was found to have a significantly higher autonomic score (4.5 ± 0.4 vs 0.9 ± 0.4).[54] Because these tests can be administered conveniently at the bedside, they may represent viable, cost effective, and clinically beneficial options to help unmask latent CAD. However, the sensitivity and specificity of the autonomic scoring system remains to be established in large, case-controlled studies.

Baseline ECG

A resting ECG can also be used to further stratify individuals according to risk. The presence of ST-T wave abnormalities had the highest odds ratio (9.27) for predicting silent ischemia on exercise testing in the Milan Study on Atherosclerosis and Diabetes (MiSAD).[55] The presence of ST-T wave abnormalities was also the only significant predictor of silent ischemia in women.[55] Rajagopalan and colleagues[33] also reported that nonspecific ST-T wave changes were strong predictors of inducible ischemia on SPECT imaging in asymptomatic diabetic patients. However, patients with ECG abnormalities were excluded from the DIAD study.[16]

Specialized Cardiovascular Tests

Following laboratory and bedside tests, the necessity for specialized cardiovascular tests such as exercise ECG, stress echocardiography, stress myocardial perfusion scanning (MPS) or electron beam computed tomography can be determined on an individual basis.

Risk stratification and exercise ECG testing

In asymptomatic patients, evaluation of CAD risk markers and risk stratification allows clinicians to determine whether exercise evaluations are necessary. Combining clinical information from risk assessment with exercise ECG test results has been reported to yield 94% sensitivity and 92% specificity.[56]

Various risk assessment tools are available to assess the risk of cardiovascular disease (CVD). A commonly used risk assessment tool published by the American College of Sports Medicine[57,58] is presented in **Tables 1** and **2**. Initial stratification uses age, CVD risk factors, and symptoms suggestive of CVD, pulmonary disease, or metabolic disease, to classify individuals as low, moderate, or high risk (see **Table 1**). CVD risk factors include family history, cigarette smoking, hypertension, dyslipidemia, impaired fasting glucose, obesity, sedentary lifestyle (positive risk factors), and high-density lipoprotein (HDL)-cholesterol (negative risk factor) (see **Table 2**).

Several other risk assessment tools are available on the Internet:

1. Framingham Risk Score: [http://hp2010.nhlbihin.net/atpiii/calculator.asp?usertype=prof]
2. The UK Prospective Diabetes Study (UKPDS): [http://www.dtu.ox.ac.uk/index.php?maindoc=/riskengine/]
3. American Diabetes Association's Diabetes PHD (Personal Health Decisions): [http://www.diabetes.org/diabetesphd/default.jsp]

The ADA's Diabetes PHD is the only tool that includes physical activity level in CVD risk assessment. In view of the established benefit of physical activity and cardiorespiratory fitness for reducing CVD risk in persons with diabetes,[6–9] the authors recommend use of the ADA's Diabetes PHD risk assessment tool.

Following risk stratification of individuals as low, moderate, or high risk, exercise ECG testing may be a cost-effective method for screening in a selected group of

Table 1	
Initial individual risk stratification	
Low risk	Men <45 years of age and women <55 years of age who are asymptomatic and meet no more than one risk factor threshold from Table 2
Moderate risk	Men ≥45 years of age and women ≥55 years of age *or* those who meet the threshold for two or more risk factors from Table 2
High risk	Individuals with one or more of the following signs and symptoms (ankle edema, palpitations or tachycardia, intermittent claudication, known heart murmur, unusual fatigue or shortness of breath with usual activities) *OR* known cardiovascular (cardiac, peripheral vascular, or cerebrovascular disease), pulmonary (chronic obstructive pulmonary disease, asthma, interstitial lung disease, cystic fibrosis), or metabolic disease (diabetes mellitus, thyroid disorders, renal, or liver disease)

Data from American College of Sports Medicine. Guidelines for exercise testing and prescription. 7th edition. Baltimore (MD): Lippincott Williams & Wilkins; 2006. p. 27.

Table 2	
Coronary artery risk factors for risk stratification	
Risk Factors	**Defining Criteria**
Positive risk factors	
Family history	Myocardial infarction, coronary revascularization, or sudden death before 55 years of age in father or other male first degree relative, or before 65 years of age in mother or other female first degree relative
Cigarette smoking	Current cigarette smoker or those who quit within the previous 6 months
Hypertension	Systolic blood pressure ≥ 140 mmHg or diastolic blood pressure ≥ 90 mmHg, confirmed by measurements on at least two separate occasions, or on anti-hypertensive medication
Dyslipidemia	Low-density lipoprotein (LDL) cholesterol > 130 mg/dL^{-1} (3.4 mmol/L^{-1}) or high-density lipoprotein (HDL) cholesterol < 40 mg/dL^{-1} (1.03 mmol/L^{-1}), or on a lipid-lowering medication. If serum cholesterol is all that is available then use > 200 mg/dL^{-1} (5.2 mmol/L^{-1}) rather than LDL > 130 mg/dL^{-1}
Impaired fasting glucose	Fasting blood glucose ≥ 100 mg/dL^{-1} (5.6 mmol/L^{-1}) confirmed by measurements on at least two separate occasions
Obesity	Body mass index >30 kg/m^2 or waist girth >102 cm for men and > 88 cm for women or waist/hip ratio: ≥ 0.95 for men and ≥ 0.86 for women
Sedentary lifestyle	Persons not participating in a regular program or not meeting the minimum physical activity recommendations of from the U.S Surgeon General's Report (accumulating 30 minutes or more of moderate physical activity on most days of the week)
Negative risk factors	
High HDL cholesterol*	> 60 mg/dl^{-1} (1.6 mmol/L^{-1})

* It is common to sum risk factors in making clinical judgments. If HDL is high, subtract one risk factor from the sum of positive risk factors, because high HDL decreases CAD risk.

From American College of Sports Medicine. Guidelines for exercise testing and prescription. 7th edition. Baltimore (MD): Lippincott Williams & Wilkins; 2006. p. 22; with permission.

individuals. In a large series of United States veterans with diabetes, although angina did not reliably accompany exercise-induced ischemia,[59] exercise-induced ST depression was associated with more cardiac events in patients with diabetes with or without associated angina, and it conferred a worse prognosis for the development of CVD.[60]

Based on a systematic review for the US Preventive Services Task Force, exercise ECG tests are not recommended to detect SMI in asymptomatic persons at low risk for CAD (eg, <10% risk of cardiac event over 10 years).[61] Because CAD-asymptomatic patients are at moderate risk for CAD events,[12] pre-exercise ECG testing is recommended for either moderate-risk patients considering a program of vigorous exercise, intensity $\geq$ 6 metabolic equivalents (METs), such as jogging, or for high-risk patients about to embark on a program of moderate or vigorous intensity exercise (**Table 3**).

Stress echocardiography

The prognostic value of stress echocardiography is well established in the general population;[62] however, its usefulness in the diabetic population is unclear. The annual event rate in diabetic patients with normal stress echocardiography ranges from 1.5% to 6.0% compared with 0.6% to 2.7% in nondiabetic patients.[62–65] Of concern, however, is the fact that although diabetic patients with a negative stress echocardiogram have a 0% event rate in the first year, event rates increase progressively from 1.8% in the third year, to 2.6% in the fourth year, and to 3.2% in the fifth year following the initial screening test. Patients with inducible ischemia in 2 or more vascular territories also have a substantially higher mortality rate at 5 years compared with those with a normal stress echo (32.8% versus 8.7% respectively).[65] This implies that although stress echocardiography cannot be used to identify low-risk diabetic patients, it is a useful tool for the identification of high-risk patients.

A submaximal test (achieving <85% of maximum heart rate) will affect the predictive value of functional cardiac testing. Although not associated with an increase in cardiac risk in normal individuals, a negative submaximal dobutamine stress echo is still associated with an elevated cardiac risk in diabetic patients.[66]

Myocardial perfusion scanning

MPS with SPECT seems to have a higher sensitivity for the detection of CAD compared with stress echocardiography.[67] An abnormal stress MPS study is strongly predictive of short- and long-term cardiac events in diabetic patients and confers a poor prognosis.[68] Several retrospective studies have confirmed that event rates

Table 3
American College of Sports Medicine recommendations for current medical examination and exercise testing prior to exercise participation

	Low Risk	Moderate Risk	High Risk
For participation in moderate-intensity exercise program	Not necessary	Not necessary	Recommended*
For participation in vigorous-intensity exercise program	Not necessary	Recommended	Recommended

* The ACSM recommends exercise testing prior to participation; this is due to the fact that the ACSM defines anyone with a metabolic disease, such as diabetes, as "high-risk." However, the American Diabetes Association does not recommend routine exercise testing in asymptomatic diabetics prior to the start of a moderate-intensity physical activity program.[9]
Data from American College of Sports Medicine. Guidelines for exercise testing and prescription. 7th edition. Baltimore (MD): Lippincott Williams & Wilkins; 2006. p. 20.

vary with the extent of inducible ischemia observed on a stress MPS study.[33,35,36,69–73] In the 22% of patients with silent ischemia in the DIAD study,[16] the strongest predictor of an abnormal stress MPS was autonomic dysfunction. This study also highlighted the inadequacy of previous ADA guidelines,[32] which would have resulted in 41% of abnormal tests being missed, and also demonstrated that previous traditional cardiac risk markers were poor predictors of myocardial perfusion abnormalities in patients with T2D.

De Lorenzo and colleagues[35] demonstrated the usefulness of stress MPS in risk stratification of asymptomatic diabetic patients. An abnormal test increased the risk of hard events by 5.4-fold and of total events by 7.4-fold. Extensive perfusion defects were associated with an 18.8-fold increase in risk of total events. Although stress MPS seems to be a promising modality for risk stratification, no outcome data with regard to early screening and intervention in an asymptomatic population exist currently.

Electron beam computed tomography

Coronary artery calcium (CAC) scoring is a simple noninvasive test that can be used to quantify the extent of coronary artery calcium, which is a reliable indicator of atherosclerosis.[74] The CAC score is a predictor of SMI and seems to be a more sensitive predictor of cardiovascular events compared with the UKPDS and the Framingham risk scores.[75]

Recommended Testing Algorithm for SMI

Anand and colleagues[75] recommended the use of a combination strategy, incorporating the use of CAC scoring and stress MPS. In this study, the severity of the CAC score had a direct relationship with the degree of ischemia elicited during a stress MPS study. The CAC score and MPS seemed to have a synergistic effect with regard to predicting event-free survival in patients with SMI. The investigators recommended that restricting MPS to only those patients with a CAC score >100 would be a good strategy because this strategy appeared to perform as well as the technique used in the DIAD study.[16] The investigators speculated that this would be a cost-effective technique if the cost of electron beam computed tomography was no more than 75% that of MPS and, as an added benefit, would also result in a reduced radiation dose per patient.

Conversely, the 2006 American College of Cardiology appropriateness criteria recommend a score of 400 as the threshold for further testing.[76] This could be a worthwhile strategy because one third of the patients in the study by Anand and colleagues[75] had a calcium score of >400, of whom approximately 28% had large ischemic deficits.

THE ECONOMICS OF SCREENING FOR SMI

Screening for SMI in asymptomatic individuals with diabetes is controversial and lacks established evidence-based guidelines. Although it is clear that diabetic patients with SMI have a poor prognosis, what is less clear is the benefit of aggressive screening methods. Diamond and colleagues[77] performed a simple "back-of-the-envelope" calculation of the cost and potential benefits of a "screen everyone" versus a "treat everyone" strategy. Using Pareto's rule, that is, 20% of patients will have 80% of the events, the total cost of screening and treating 14 million diabetic patients would be approximately $13.3 billion (screen everyone) compared with $10.1 billion (treat everyone). The average cost per life year would be $15,224 versus $9,249.

It is also important to note that screening alone does not treat anyone, and, because the tests themselves are not infallible, it would lower the effects of the intervention.

Most studies advocating screening, however, are tainted by the caveat that outcome studies have yet to be performed to demonstrate the effectiveness of a screening strategy, that is, a trial to prove the superiority of a "screen everyone" strategy versus a "treat everyone" strategy. Performing such a study would be a daunting process. Given the small difference in projected outcome (ie, 7% versus 7.6% for conditional testing over 5 years), a trial to prove the superiority of "screen everyone" over "treat everyone" would need 80,000 subjects followed for 5 years, assuming zero dropouts.

In consideration of the prohibitive costs, perhaps the best strategy in these patients may be to avoid screening unless there is a high index of clinical suspicion, and instead treat all concerned. If there is concern regarding the safety of the patient with regard to an exercise-based intervention, the treating physician could choose to have the patient enroll in a clinically supervised program of cardiac rehabilitation as a first step in the process. Because the risks associated with physical activity drop significantly following acclimatization to exercise, after an initial bout of cardiac rehabilitation, a patient can be transitioned to an independent or group-based exercise program. However, cardiac rehabilitation for asymptomatic diabetic patients is not currently covered by Medicare, and thus would impose a significant cost burden on the patient.

SUMMARY

CAD is a major cause of morbidity and mortality in persons with diabetes. Exercise is an important cornerstone in the treatment and management of diabetes but is also associated with a heightened risk of sudden cardiac death in those with occult CAD. Before beginning a physical activity program that involves anything greater than moderate-intensity exercise (eg, more strenuous than brisk walking), consideration should be given to screening asymptomatic persons with diabetes for SMI. Screening can be accomplished by using risk stratification models and simple bedside tests coupled with specialized cardiovascular testing modalities.

The final decision as to whether or not to screen for occult CAD in asymptomatic diabetic patients rests with the clinician and must be carefully examined on a case-by-case basis. A careful review of systems and clinical examination is essential because combining those with a functional test such as an exercise ECG displays impressive diagnostic yields for SMI (94% sensitivity and 92% specificity),[57] which in turn could help set the stage for an aggressive primary or secondary prevention and risk reduction program. Several investigators are in agreement that there seems to be no need to pursue an aggressive testing algorithm in asymptomatic diabetic patients who intend to pursue an exercise program of moderate intensity and that pre-exercise screening could be of some use in ensuring the safety of those individuals looking to pursue a high-intensity exercise program.

REFERENCES

1. Blendea MC, McFarlane SI, Isenovic ER, et al. Heart disease in diabetic patients. Curr Diab Rep 2003;3:223–9.
2. Bonow RO, Bohannon N, Hazzard W. Risk stratification in coronary artery disease and special populations [review]. Am J Med 1996;101:17S–22S.
3. Dorman JS, Laporte RE, Kuller LH, et al. The Pittsburgh insulin-dependent diabetes mellitus (IDDM) morbidity and mortality study. Mortality results. Diabetes 1984;33:271–6.
4. Laing SP, Swerdlow AJ, Slater SD, et al. Mortality from heart disease in a cohort of 23,000 patients with insulin-treated diabetes. Diabetologia 2003;46:760–5.

5. Moss SE, Klein R, Klein BE. Cause-specific mortality in a population-based study of diabetes. Am J Public Health 1991;81:1158–62.
6. Church TS, LaMonte MJ, Barlow CE, et al. Cardiorespiratory fitness and body mass index as predictors of cardiovascular disease mortality among men with diabetes. Arch Intern Med 2005;165:2114–20.
7. Wing RR, Jakicic J, Neiberg R, et al. Fitness, fatness, and cardiovascular risk factors in type 2 diabetes: look ahead study. Med Sci Sports Exerc 2007;39:2107–16.
8. American Diabetes Association. Diabetes mellitus and exercise. Diabetes Care 2002;25:S64–8.
9. Sigal RJ, Kenny GP, Wasserman DH, et al. Physical activity/exercise and type 2 diabetes. A consensus statement from the American Diabetes Association. Diabetes Care 2006;29:1433–8.
10. Bax JJ, Bonow RO, Tschope D, et al. on behalf of the Global Dialogue Group for the Evaluation of Cardiovascular Risk in Patients With Diabetes. The potential of myocardial perfusion scintigraphy for risk stratification of asymptomatic patients with type 2 diabetes. J Am Coll Cardiol 2006;48:754–60.
11. Miller TD, Redberg RF, Wackers FJT. Screening asymptomatic diabetic patients for coronary artery disease. Why not? J Am Coll Cardiol 2006;48:761–4.
12. Bax JJ, Young LH, Frye RL, et al. Screening for coronary artery disease in patients with diabetes. Diabetes Care 2007;30:2729–36.
13. Multiple Risk Factor Intervention Trial Research Group. Exercise electrocardiogram and coronary heart disease mortality in the Multiple Risk Factor Intervention Trial. Am J Cardiol 1985;55:16–24.
14. Rutter MK, Wahid ST, McComb JM, et al. Significance of silent ischemia and microalbuminuria in predicting coronary events in asymptomatic patients with type 2 diabetes. J Am Coll Cardiol 2002;40:56–61.
15. Fornengo P, Bosio A, Epifani G, et al. Prevalence of silent myocardial ischemia in new-onset middle-aged Type 2 diabetic patients without other cardiovascular risk factors. Diabetes Med 2006;23:775–9.
16. Wackers FJ, Young LH, Inzucchi SE, et al. Detection of Ischemia in Asymptomatic Diabetics Investigators. Detection of silent myocardial ischemia in asymptomatic diabetic subjects: the DIAD study. Diabetes Care 2004;27:1954–61.
17. Janand-Delenne B, Savin B, Habib G, et al. Silent myocardial ischemia in patients with diabetes: who to screen. Diabetes Care 1999;22:1396–400.
18. BARI Investigators. Influence of diabetes on 5-year mortality and morbidity in a randomized trial comparing CABG and PTCA in patients with multivessel disease: the Bypass Angioplasty Revascularization Investigation (BARI). Circulation 1997;96:1761–9.
19. BARI Investigators. Seven-year outcome in the Bypass Angioplasty Revascularization Investigation (BARI) by treatment and diabetic status. J Am Coll Cardiol 2000;35:1122–9.
20. Larsen J, Brekke M, Sandvik L, et al. Silent coronary atheromatosis in type 1 diabetic patients and its relation to long-term glycemic control. Diabetes 2002;51:2637–41.
21. Wackers FJ, Chyun DA, Young LH, et al. Detection of Ischemia in Asymptomatic Diabetics (DIAD) Investigators. Resolution of asymptomatic myocardial ischemia in patients with type 2 diabetes in the Detection of Ischemia in Asymptomatic Diabetics (DIAD) study. Diabetes Care 2007;30:2892–8.
22. Faglia E, Manuela M, Antonella Q, et al. Risk reduction of cardiac events by screening of unknown asymptomatic coronary artery disease in subjects with

type 2 diabetes mellitus at high cardiovascular risk: an open-label randomized pilot study. Am Heart J 2005;149:e1–6.

23. Sorajja P, Chareonthaitawee P, Rajagopalan N, et al. Improved survival in asymptomatic diabetic patients with high-risk SPECT imaging treated with coronary artery bypass grafting. Circulation 2005;112(9 Suppl):I311–6.

24. Kohl HW, Powell KE, Gordon NF, et al. Physical activity, physical fitness, and sudden cardiac death. Epidemiol Rev 1992;14:37–57.

25. Paterson DJ. Antiarrhythmic mechanisms during exercise. J Appl Physiol 1996; 80:1853–62.

26. Willich SN, Maclure M, Mittleman M, et al. Sudden cardiac death: support for a role of triggering in causation. Circulation 1993;87:1442–50.

27. Sexton PT, Walsh J, Jamrozik K, et al. Risk factors for sudden unexpected cardiac death in Tasmanian men. Aust N Z J Med 1997;27:45–50.

28. Lemaitre RN, Siscovick DS, Raghunathan TE, et al. Leisure-time physical activity and the risk of primary cardiac arrest. Arch Intern Med 1999;159:686–90.

29. Erbs S, Linke A, Hambrecht R. Effects of exercise training on mortality in patients with coronary heart disease. Coron Artery Dis 2006;17:219–25.

30. Hambrecht R, Walther C, Möbius-Winkler S, et al. Percutaneous coronary angioplasty compared with exercise training in patients with stable coronary artery disease: a randomized trial. Circulation 2004;109:1371–8.

31. Kendziorra K, Walther C, Foerster M, et al. Changes in myocardial perfusion due to physical exercise in patients with stable coronary artery disease. Eur J Nucl Med Mol Imaging 2005;32:813–9.

32. American Diabetes Association. Consensus development conference on the diagnosis of coronary heart disease in people with diabetes. Diabetes Care 1998;21:1551–9.

33. Rajagopalan N, Miller TD, Hodge DO, et al. Identifying high risk asymptomatic diabetic patients who are candidates for screening stress single photon emission computed tomography imaging. J Am Coll Cardiol 2005;45:43–9.

34. Scognamiglio R, Negut C, Ramondo A, et al. Detection of coronary artery disease in asymptomatic patients with type 2 diabetes mellitus. J Am Coll Cardiol 2006; 47:65–71.

35. De Lorenzo A, Lima RS, Siqueira-Filho AG, et al. Prevalence and prognostic value of perfusion defects detected by stress technetium-99m sestamibi myocardial perfusion single-photon emission computed tomography in asymptomatic patients with diabetes mellitus and no known coronary artery disease. Am J Cardiol 2002;90(8):827–32.

36. Giri S, Shaw LJ, Murthy DR, et al. Impact of diabetes on the risk stratification using stress single-photon emission computed tomography myocardial perfusion imaging in patients with symptoms suggestive of coronary artery disease. Circulation 2002;105(1):32–40.

37. Sultan A, Piot C, Mariano-Goulart D, et al. Risk factors for silent myocardial ischemia in high-risk type 1 diabetic patients. Diabetes Care 2004;27(7):1745–57.

38. Akasaka T, Yoshida K, Hozumi T, et al. Retinopathy identifies marked restriction of coronary flow reserve in patients with diabetes mellitus. J Am Coll Cardiol 1997; 30:935–41.

39. Abbott RD, Donahue RP, Kannel WB, et al. The impact of diabetes on survival following myocardial infarction in men vs women: the Framingham Study. JAMA 1988;260:3456–60.

40. Kloner RA. Erectile dysfunction: the new harbinger for major adverse cardiac events in the diabetic patient. J Am Coll Cardiol 2008;51:2051–2.

41. Ma RC, So WY, Yang X, et al. Erectile dysfunction predicts coronary heart disease in type 2 diabetes. J Am Coll Cardiol 2008;51(21):2045–50.

42. Ward RC, Weiner J, Taillon LA, et al. Comparison of findings on stress myocardial perfusion imaging in men with versus without erectile dysfunction and without prior heart disease. Am J Cardiol 2008;101(4):502–5.

43. Rutter MK, McComb JM, Brady S, et al. Silent myocardial ischemia and microalbuminuria in asymptomatic subjects with non-insulin-dependent diabetes mellitus. Am J Cardiol 1999;83(1):27–31.

44. Papaioannou GI, Seip RL, Grey NJ, et al. Brachial artery reactivity in asymptomatic patients with type 2 diabetes mellitus and microalbuminuria (from the Detection of Ischemia in Asymptomatic Diabetics-brachial artery reactivity study). Am J Cardiol 2004;94(3):294–9.

45. Mann JF, Gerstein HC, Pogue J, et al. Renal insufficiency as a predictor of cardiovascular outcomes and the impact of ramipril: the HOPE randomized trial. Ann Intern Med 2001;134:629–36.

46. Araz M, Celen Z, Akdemir I, et al. Frequency of silent myocardial ischemia in type 2 diabetic patients and the relation with poor glycemic control. Acta Diabetol 2004;41(2):38–43.

47. Milan Study on Atherosclerosis and Diabetes (MISAD Group). Prevalence of unrecognized silent myocardial ischemia and its association with atherosclerotic risk factors in non-insulin dependent diabetes mellitus. Am J Cardiol 1997;79: 134–9.

48. Naka M, Hiramatsu K, Aizawa T, et al. Silent myocardial ischemia in patients with non-insulin-dependent diabetes mellitus as judged by treadmill exercise testing and coronary angiography. Am Heart J 1992;123(1):46–53.

49. Earle KA, Mishra M, Morocutti A, et al. Microalbuminuria as a marker of silent myocardial ischaemia in IDDM patients. Diabetologia 1996;39:854–6.

50. Intensive blood-glucose control with sulphonylureas or insulin compared with conventional treatment and risk of complications in patients with type 2 diabetes (UKPDS 33): UK Prospective Diabetes Study (UKPDS) Group. Lancet 1998;352: 837–53.

51. Laakso M. Hyperglycemia and cardiovascular disease in type 2 diabetes. Diabetes 1999;48:937–42.

52. Doobay AV, Anand SS. Sensitivity and specificity of the ankle-brachial index to predict future cardiovascular outcomes: a systematic review. Arterioscler Thromb Vasc Biol 2005;25(7):1463–9.

53. Hiatt WR. Medical treatment of peripheral arterial disease and claudication. N Engl J Med 2001;344:1608–21.

54. Baxter CG, Boon NA, Walker JD. Detection of silent myocardial ischemia in asymptomatic diabetic subjects: the DIAD study. Diabetes Care 2005;28(3):756–7.

55. MiSAD investigators. Prevalence of unrecognized silent myocardial ischemia and its association with atherosclerotic risk factors in noninsulin-dependent diabetes mellitus. Milan Study on Atherosclerosis and Diabetes (MiSAD) Group. Am J Cardiol 1997;79(2):134–9.

56. Do D, West JA, Morise A, et al. A consensus approach to diagnosing coronary artery disease based on clinical and exercise test data. Chest 1997;111:1742–9.

57. American College of Sports Medicine. Guidelines for exercise testing and prescription. 7th edition. Baltimore (MD): Lippincott Williams & Wilkins; 2006. p. 19–35.

58. Harris GD, White RD. Exercise stress testing in patients with type 2 diabetes: when are asymptomatic patients screened? Clin Diabetes 2007;25:126–30.

59. Nesto RW, Phillips RT, Kett KG, et al. Angina and exertional myocardial ischemia in diabetic and nondiabetic patients: assessment by exercise thallium scintigraphy [published erratum appears in Ann Intern Med 1988;108:646]. Ann Intern Med 1988;108:170–5.

60. Callaham PR, Froelicher VF, Klein J, et al. Exercise-induced silent ischemia: age, diabetes mellitus, previous myocardial infarction and prognosis. J Am Coll Cardiol 1989;14:1175–80.

61. Fowler-Brown A, Pignone M, Pletcher M, et al. Exercise tolerance testing to screen for coronary heart disease: a systematic review for the technical support for the U.S. Preventive Service Task Force. Ann Intern Med 2004;140:W9–24.

62. McCully RB, Roger VL, Mahoney DW, et al. Outcome after normal exercise echocardiography and predictors of subsequent cardiac events: follow-up of 1325 patients. J Am Coll Cardiol 1998;31:144–9.

63. Anand DV, Lim E, Lahiri A, et al. The role of non-invasive imaging in the risk stratification of asymptomatic diabetic subjects. Eur Heart J 2006;27(8):905–12.

64. Kamalesh M, Matorin R, Sawada S. Prognostic value of negative stress echocardiographic study in diabetic patients. Am Heart J 2002;143:163–8.

65. Elhendy A, Arruda AM, Mahoney DM, et al. Prognostic stratification of diabetic patients by exercise echocardiography. J Am Coll Cardiol 2001;37:1551–7.

66. Patel SJ, Srivastava A, Lingam N, et al. Prognostic significance of submaximal negative dobutamine stress echocardiography: a 3-year follow-up study. Cardiol J 2008;15(3):237–44.

67. Schinkel AFL, Bax JJ, Geleijnse ML, et al. Non-invasive evaluation of ischemic heart disease: myocardial perfusion imaging or stress echocardiography. Eur Heart J 2003;24:789–800.

68. Felsher J, Meissner MD, Hakki AH, et al. Exercise thallium imaging in patients with diabetes mellitus. Prognostic implications. Arch Intern Med 1987;147:313–7.

69. Vanzetto G, Halimi S, Hammoud T, et al. Prediction of cardiovascular events in clinically selected high-risk NIDDM patients: prognostic value of exercise stress test and thallium-201 single-photon emission computed tomography. Diabetes Care 1999;22:19–26.

70. Kang X, Berman DS, Lewin HC, et al. Incremental prognostic value of myocardial perfusion single photon emission computed tomography in patients with diabetes mellitus. Am Heart J 1999;138:1025–32.

71. Schinkel AFL, Elhendy A, Van Domburg RT, et al. Prognostic value of dobutamine–atropine stress myocardial perfusion imaging in patients with diabetes. Diabetes Care 2002;25:1637–43.

72. Zellweger MJ, Hachamovitch R, Kang X, et al. Prognostic relevance of symptoms versus evidence of coronary artery disease in diabetic patients. Eur Heart J 2004;25:543–50.

73. Cosson E, Guimfack M, Paries J, et al. Prognosis for coronary stenoses in patients with diabetes and silent myocardial ischemia. Diabetes Care 2003;26:1313–4.

74. Rumberger JA, Simons DB, Fitzpatrick LA, et al. Coronary artery calcium area by electron beam computed tomography and coronary atherosclerotic plaque area: a histopathologic correlative study. Circulation 1995;92:2157–62.

75. Anand DV, Lim E, Hopkins D, et al. Risk stratification in uncomplicated type 2 diabetes: prospective evaluation of the combined use of coronary artery calcium imaging and selective myocardial perfusion scintigraphy. Eur Heart J 2006;27(6):713–21.

76. Hendel RC, Patel MR, Kramer CM, et al. ACCF/ACR/SCCT/SCMR/ASNC/NASCI/ SCAI/SIR 2006 appropriateness criteria for cardiac computed tomography and cardiac magnetic resonance imaging: a report of the American College of Cardiology Foundation Quality Strategic Directions Committee Appropriateness Criteria Working Group, American College of Radiology, Society of Cardiovascular Computed Tomography, Society for Cardiovascular Magnetic Resonance, American Society of Nuclear Cardiology, North American Society for Cardiac Imaging, Society for Cardiovascular Angiography and Interventions, and Society of Interventional Radiology. J Am Coll Cardiol 2006;48(7):1475–97.

77. Diamond GA, Kaul S, Shah PK. Screen testing cardiovascular prevention in asymptomatic diabetic patients. J Am Coll Cardiol 2007;49(19):1915–7.

Exercise for Prevention of Obesity and Diabetes in Children and Adolescents

Anthony McCall, MD, PhD[a],*, Ramona Raj, MD[b]

KEYWORDS

- Obesity prevention • Diabetes prevention • Obesity • Diabetes
- Childhood obesity prevention • Type 2 diabetes prevention
- Childhood diabetes prevention

In preindustrial times, our ability to store fat undoubtedly led ironically to the "survival of the fittest." In the Paleolithic and Mesolithic eras, conditions of feast or famine required the ability to store fat in times of need. Hunting and foraging resulted in avolatile food supply and required constant human movement. Even as humans transitioned to an agricultural age in the Neolithic period, these preindustrial societies required large energy expenditures in animal husbandry and plant cultivation in the absence of mechanization.

In today's world of labor stratification, declining physical exercise, and easy access to energy-dense foods, or otherwise what is often termed an "obesogenic" environment, the model of what was once advantageous to survival is no longer the case. Heart disease is the leading cause of mortality in the United States, with cerebrovascular disease and diabetes well within the top 10 causes of death.[1] All 3 of these have been linked to obesity and the metabolic syndrome.

Obesity often predisposes patients to type 2 diabetes, hypertension, and dyslipidemia or the metabolic syndrome largely through the production of increased free fatty acids and adipokines by the increased amounts of adipose tissue. With increased lipolysis in obesity, there is increased free fatty acid production, which interferes with insulin receptor signaling and leads to decreased glucose transport, often referred to as lipotoxicity. Increased fatty acids ultimately result in activating protein kinase C (through increased fatty Acyl-CoA and diacylglycerols), and, in turn, protein kinase C serine phosphorylates the insulin receptor, interfering with insulin signal

[a] Division of Endocrinology, Department of Internal Medicine, University of Virginia Health System, PO Box 801407, Charlottesville, VA 22908, USA
[b] Division of Endocrinology, Department of Internal Medicine, University of Virginia Health System, PO Box 801408, Charlottesville, VA 22908-1408, USA
* Corresponding author.
E-mail address: alm3j@virgina.edu (A. McCall).

Clin Sports Med 28 (2009) 393–421
doi:10.1016/j.csm.2009.03.001   sportsmed.theclinics.com
0278-5919/09/$ – see front matter © 2009 Elsevier Inc. All rights reserved.

transduction. Increased free fatty acids also impair phosphoinositide (PI)-3 kinase activation in response to insulin, which results in downstream decreased activity of glucose transporter-4 (GLUT4), an important insulin-sensitive glucose transporter in muscle and fat. In an obese state, some adipokines, proteins such as tumor necrosis factor alpha (TNF-α), or cytokines such as interleukin-6 (IL-6) are elevated, whereas adiponectin, an insulin-sensitizing adipokine, is low. Adipokines inhibit insulin action and contribute to proinflammatory effects, insulin resistance, and endothelial dysfunction. This eventually results in an increased risk for myocardial infarction and stroke.

OBESITY PREVALENCE

The fact that obesity is the largest epidemic of our times is confirmed by the most recent NHANES data for 2005 to 2000 indicating that the prevalence of obesity among adults is 34%.[2] This is in contrast to just 20 years ago, when age-adjusted obesity rates in NHANES III 1988 to 1994 were 23%. A visual representation of the US distribution of obesity can be seen in **Fig. 1**, with only 1 state (Colorado) currently with a prevalence of adult obesity less than 20% and most of the country with a prevalence of obesity greater than 25%.

Adult obesity is also reflected in rates of childhood overweight and obesity. NHANES data for the combined years of 2003 to 2006 indicate that 16.3% of children and adolescents aged 2 to 19 years are obese, defined as at or above the 95th percentile of the 2000 body mass index (BMI)-for age growth charts.[3] This is compared with about 5% in NHANES III data from 1988 to 1994. This is even more striking when considering the number of children at risk for obesity currently. NHANES survey data from 2003 to 2006 find that 32% of the children in the United States are overweight, defined as at or above the 85th percentile of the 2000 BMI-for age growth charts. **Fig. 2** illustrates the trend in overweight rates for selected years from 1976 to 2004.

Obesity Trends* Among U.S. Adults
BRFSS, 1990, 1998, 2007
(*BMI ≥30, or about 30 lbs. overweight for 5'4" person)

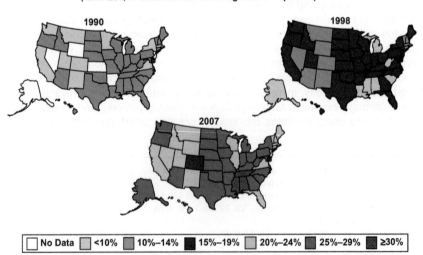

| | No Data | <10% | 10%–14% | 15%–19% | 20%–24% | 25%–29% | ≥30% |

Fig. 1. Obesity trends. (*Adapted from* Centers for Disease Control. U.S. Obesity Trends 1985–2007. Available at: http://www.cdc.gov/nccdphp/dnpa/obesity/trend/maps/#PDF.)

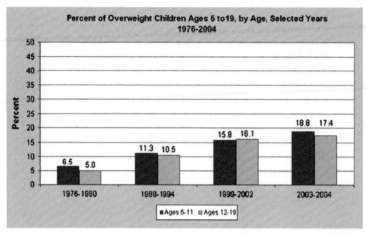

Fig. 2. Overweight trends for children. (*Courtesy of* Child Trends Data Bank, Washington, DC; with permission.)

The rise in obesity has not been confined to the United States. According to a pooled analysis of worldwide data in 2005, 23.2% of the world's population is overweight, with a BMI of 25 kg/m² or greater. About 8% of the world's population is obese, with a BMI at or greater than 30 kg/m².[4] Although the prevalence of overweight and obesity was higher in developed countries than that in developing countries (35.2% vs 19.6% and 20.3% vs 6%, respectively) the larger population in developing countries results in an overall larger global population being affected. This is also supported by World Health Organization (WHO) data (refer to **Fig. 3**). If current trends continue, the WHO predicts that there will be 2.3 billion overweight adults in the world by 2015, and more than 700 million of them will be obese.

In terms of worldwide childhood obesity, defining overweight as a weight-for-height greater than 2 standard deviations above the National Center for Health Statistics/WHO international reference median, one study found that the global prevalence of overweight was 3.3% in children.[5] Although childhood malnourishment is still a critical concern in many countries, the number of overweight children is growing, with the highest overweight prevalence rates in the Americas, Europe, and the Middle East, according to data from the International Obesity Task Force (**Fig. 4**).

OBESITY PREVENTION IN ADULTS

Preventing obesity in adults has largely been studied in selected populations or in the context of preventing diabetes. A small randomized, controlled trial (n = 40) known as the Health Hunters pilot study focused on young women with at least 1 obese parent.[6] The study found that an intervention dedicated to improving physical activity and diet resulted in weight stability compared with the weight gain in the control group after 1 year. Another randomized controlled trial studied older women.[7] This trial was larger (n = 173) and involved overweight, obese, postmenopausal women who were randomized to either 45 minutes of moderate-intensity physical exercise 5 d/wk or the control group. The exercise group had a significant decrease in body weight (-1.4 kg), total body fat (-1.0%) as studied by dual-energy x-ray absorptiometry (DXA), intra-abdominal fat (-8.6 g/cm²), and subcutaneous abdominal fat (-28.8 g/cm²) as studied by computed tomography at 1 year. These studies were small and

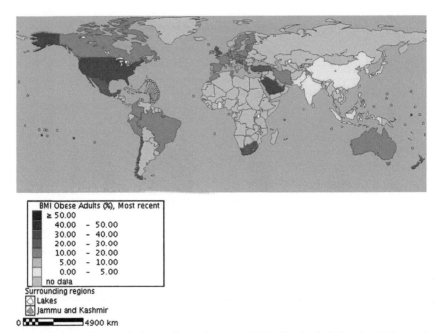

Fig. 3. Global Prevalence of obesity, from the WHO 2005. Obesity is defined as BMI equal to or greater than 30%. (*Courtesy of* the World Health Organization. Global database on body mass index. Available at http://www.who.int/bmi/index.jsp.)

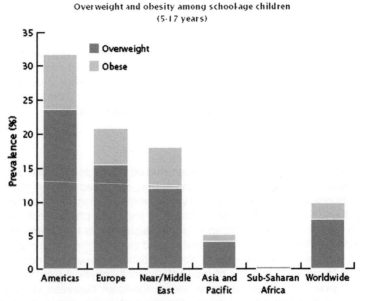

Fig. 4. Worldwide childhood obesity prevalence. (*From* International Diabetes Foundation. Diabetes atlas. 2nd edition. Brussels: International Diabetes Foundation; 2003; with permission. Available at: www.eatlas.idf.org.)

lacked long-term follow-up data but suggested that interventions involving diet and exercise could be useful in preventing obesity in women.

DIABETES PREVENTION IN ADULTS

The Finnish Diabetes Prevention study was designed to determine if type 2 diabetes can be prevented by behavioral lifestyle modifications, emphasizing diet and exercise.[8] The study enrolled 523 middle-aged patients with a BMI at or greater than 25 kg/m^2, with impaired glucose tolerance as determined by an oral glucose tolerance test (OGTT). It used the older 1985 WHO definition of diabetes as a fasting blood glucose greater than 140 mg/dL. Subjects were either randomized to a control group, with some general information on diet and exercise, or the intervention group, who received detailed individualized diet and exercise information. The intervention group also received individual nutritionist sessions and weight training sessions. The goals of the lifestyle intervention included 5% body weight loss, 30% decrease in total fat intake with a 10% decrease in saturated fats, increased fiber, and moderate exercise for at least 30 minutes daily. After 2 years of enrollment in the study, the intervention group had a mean 3.5-kg loss in weight compared with a 0.8-kg loss in the control group. Only 27 patients were diagnosed with diabetes in the intervention group compared with 59 in the control group at the end of the study. The risk of diabetes was thus reduced in the intervention group by 58% ($P<.001$). In fact, none of the patients in either the intervention group (49) or the control group (15) who reached 4 out of the 5 goals developed diabetes. This suggests that individualized lifestyle interventions can decrease the risk of diabetes by 58% and almost 100% in those patients meeting the goals of this intervention. After 3 years of follow-up, the intervention group had a 36% decrease in the risk of diabetes.

The Finnish Diabetes Prevention Study significantly reduced cardiometabolic risk through an effective intervention with relatively modest goals. The long-term data from the Finnish Diabetes Study indicated that a difference between the groups remained 7 years after the end of the study, with incidence rates for the intervention group at 4·3 (95% confidence interval [CI], 3·4–5·4) and for the control at 7·4 (6·1–8·9) per 100 person years.[9] The cumulative incidence of diabetes at year 6 was 23% in the intervention group and 38% in the control group, with an absolute risk reduction of 15% (7·2–23·2). The relative risk reduction was 43%, which was less than the 58% seen during the original study. As expected, several subjects went on to develop diabetes over the follow-up period of 7 years. The results of the original Finnish Diabetes Prevention Study were convincing enough to lead to a national diabetes prevention program that has been implemented in Finland, which initially identifies high-risk individuals with a simple, validated risk-score questionnaire.[10]

The DPP was another large randomized, controlled trial in adults, aimed at identifying effective methods for the prevention of diabetes.[11] The study had 3234 overweight or obese subjects, with impaired fasting glucose and impaired glucose tolerance, who were randomized to standard lifestyle changes, standard lifestyle changes and metformin, or intensive lifestyle changes. Standard lifestyle changes involved provision of written information and 1 20- to 30-minute individual session annually. By comparison, the intensive lifestyle arm involved 16 individualized sessions, with goals to decrease weight by 7% through a low-fat diet and 150 minutes of moderately intense physical activity per week (mostly walking). About 74% of the subjects in the intensive arm were able to meet the goals for physical activity at 24 weeks, and 54%, at the last visit. **Fig. 5** offers a comparison in MET (metabolic equivalent of task) hours per week between the lifestyle, metformin, and placebo groups in

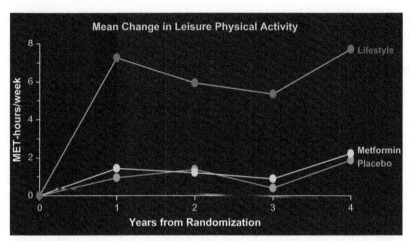

Fig. 5. Change in physical activity in DPP trial. (*Courtesy of* the Diabetes Prevention Program, Rockville, MD. Available at: http://www.bsc.gwu.edu/dpp/slides.htmlvdoc.)

terms of physical activity achieved. In fact, the results were so overwhelmingly favorable for the intensive lifestyle group that it became necessary to terminate the study a year early. Average weight loss was 0.1 kg for the standard lifestyle group, 2.1 kg for the metformin group, and 5.6 kg for the intensive lifestyle group, with an average follow-up of 2.8 years (**Fig. 6**). The incidence of diabetes was 31% lower in the metformin group and 58% lower in the intensive lifestyle changes group compared with the standard lifestyle changes group. Interestingly, this contrast was even greater in patients older than 60 years of age on subgroup analysis (**Fig. 7**).

The DPP further emphasized the importance of diet and exercise in the prevention of diabetes by suggesting that it was more effective than even the first-line pharmacologic treatment of diabetes, metformin. In addition, in the posttreatment analysis of this study of the 1274 participants who had not developed diabetes, a repeat OGTT

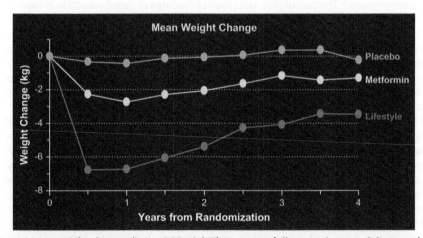

Fig. 6. Mean weight change during DPP trial. The average follow-up time was 2.8 years, that is, the number of participants decreased during the course of the study. (*Courtesy of* the Diabetes Prevention Program, Rockville, MD. Available at: http://www.bsc.gwu.edu/dpp/slides.htmlvdoc.)

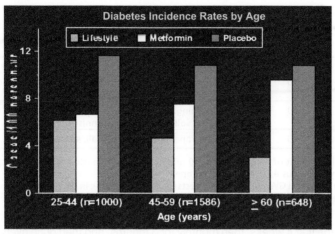

Fig. 7. Effectiveness of lifestyle compared with metformin in elderly. (*Courtesy of* the Diabetes Prevention Program, Rockville, MD. Available at: http://www.bsc.gwu.edu/dpp/slides.htmlvdoc.)

was performed after a washout period of 1 to 2 weeks off metformin.[12] After the washout, diabetes was diagnosed more in the metformin group than before the washout, suggesting that metformin was not truly preventing diabetes but instead really pretreating it. Although the authors state that there was still a 25% reduction compared with placebo in this group, we do not know if the reduction may have been smaller if they had used a longer washout period. It may be debated whether metformin alters the progression of the underlying disease process or is instead a pretreatment.

By contrast, exercise has been shown to clearly increase insulin sensitivity and alter the pathophysiological conditions underlying the development of diabetes. Exercise through muscle contractions increases translocation of GLUT4 transporters to the cell surface, increasing peripheral uptake of glucose. Exercise-mediated effects are insensitive to inhibitors of PI 3-kinase unlike insulin-mediated GLUT4 transport. In fact, exercise increases the amount of GLUT4 transporters locating to the cell surface in response to the same dose of insulin. Exercise also activates AMP (adenosine monophosphate)-dependent kinase (AMPK), which lowers Acyl-CoA levels and increases insulin signal transduction. Many of these effects of exercise can be seen independent of weight loss.

The benefits of exercise for adults in preventing diabetes are apparent in the recent publication of the 20-year follow-up data of the Da Qing Study.[13] In 1986, 577 adults with impaired glucose tolerance at 33 clinics in Da Qing City, China, were randomized by clinic site to a control, diet, exercise, or diet plus exercise group.[14] The diet group participants were prescribed a diet containing 25 to 30 kcal/kg body weight (105–126 kJ/kg), 55% to 65% carbohydrate, 10% to 15% protein, and 25% to 30%. They and were encouraged to increase their vegetable intake and decrease their alcohol and simple sugar intake. Overweight subjects (BMI $\geq$ to 25 kg/m^2) were encouraged to decrease their calorie intake to lose weight until they reached a BMI of at least 23 kg/m^2. Patients received individualized counseling sessions with their physician and periodic small group counseling sessions. The exercise group was encouraged to increase leisure exercise by at least 1 unit a day, with 2 units for younger subjects. Units varied from 5 minutes of very strenuous exercise to 30 minutes of mild exercise (refer to **Table 1**). The exercise group also had periodic small group sessions, once

Table 1
Units of activity

Intensity	Time (min)	Exercise
Mild	30	Slow walking, traveling by bus, shopping, housecleaning
Moderate	20	Faster walking or walking down stairs, cycling, doing heavy laundry, ballroom dancing (slow)
Strenuous	10	Slow running, climbing stairs, disco dancing for the elderly, playing volleyball or table tennis
Very strenuous	5	Jumping rope, playing basketball, swimming

Each example is 1 unit of activity that is, 30 min of mild exercise (slow walking) is equivalent to 5 min of very strenuous exercise (jumping rope)
Data from Pan XR, Li GW, Hu YH, et al. Effects of diet and exercise in preventing NIDDM in people with impaired glucose tolerance. The Da Qing IGT and Diabetes Study. Diabetes Care 1997;20:37–44.

weekly for the first 4 weeks, then monthly for 3 months, and then once every 3 months for the remainder of the study. The diet plus exercise group received both of these interventions. The 6-year data indicated that the cumulative diabetes incidence was 43% in the intervention group (with no significant difference between diet, exercise, or diet and exercise interventions) and 66% in the control group. The number needed to treat to prevent 1 case of diabetes was 6, and the intervention group after multivariate analysis had a 43% lower incidence of developing diabetes than the control group (hazard rate ratio, 0.57; 95% CI, 0.41–0.81).

During the 20-year follow-up, the cumulative diabetes incidence was 80% in the intervention group and 93% in the control. In addition, the participants in the intervention had an average of 3 to 6 fewer years with diabetes. However, it must be noted that the subjects in the intervention arm were 2 years younger on average at baseline, although there were no differences in other baseline characteristics, such as lipids, BMI, and fasting glucose. In 2006, there was no difference in the surviving participants in the intervention and control groups in terms of total calorie intake or the amount of leisure time physical activity when they were questioned about the preceding 1 year. The Da Qing follow-up study illustrates that the long-term effects of exercise can delay the progression to diabetes by a few years, although it may not prevent diabetes without sustained lifestyle changes, including continued exercise.

These are some of the trials that have led the American Diabetes Association to recommend for adults modest weight loss (5%–10% body weight) and regular physical activity through behavioral changes in lifestyle to prevent diabetes. However, one of the greatest difficulties that have been observed in weight loss trials has been a tendency to regain weight in long-term follow-up. Studies have shown that after being treated for 20 to 30 weeks with behavioral intervention adult subjects typically regain about 30% to 35% of their lost weight in the year following treatment.[15] Often at 5 years, these patients return to their baseline weights. In addition, data from studies of specific populations cannot always be extrapolated to a large diverse population base. When patients are enrolled in studies to lose weight, they are often given more structured individualized attention than resources allow in a community setting. In addition, many patients who are enrolled in studies are often either self-selected or selected through the study recruiters with an unintentional bias toward compliance.

Further obstacles to sustained weight loss and increased physical activity may be that this involves permanently altering behavioral patterns that are often established in childhood. If public health goals are to prevent obesity and type 2 diabetes, targeting the prevention of obesity in adulthood may be too late considering that one-third of adults in the United States are already obese. In fact, many adults learn about lifestyle changes only after being diagnosed with illnesses such as type 2 diabetes. Although the metabolic syndrome in children remains controversial,[16] most of the children who are obese tend to mature into obese adults. This has particular resonance in preadolescence and adolescence. A longitudinal study demonstrated that two-third of the children who are obese at the age of 10 years and older are likely to become obese as adults.[17] The prevention of obesity in childhood would protect the advances that have been made toward decreasing human morbidity and mortality.

THE RISKS OF CHILDHOOD OBESITY AND METABOLIC SYNDROME

The risks of childhood obesity are not limited to ensuing adult obesity. A recent study of 439 obese children considered several factors similar to those that define metabolic syndrome in adults.[18] Compared with a group of nonobese siblings, a significantly larger percentage of the obese subjects were found to have systolic/diastolic blood pressures (BPs) above the 95th percentile, triglycerides above the 95 percentile, high-density lipoprotein (HDL) levels less than the 5th percentile, and impaired glucose tolerance. Surrogate markers of inflammation such as C-reactive protein (CRP) and IL-6 were also elevated in the obese subjects. Adiponectin was decreased as can be expected in insulin-resistant individuals. In fact, in the 2-year follow-up of 77 of the study subjects, 8 out the initial 34 who met the authors' criteria for metabolic syndrome developed type 2 diabetes. Another cross-sectional study examined the quality of life of children through questionnaires and found that obese children and adolescents reported a significant impairment in all aspects that were examined (including physical, psychosocial, emotional, social, and school functioning) in comparison with healthy children and adolescents.[19] In fact, the authors remark in their comments that "The likelihood of an obese child or adolescent having impaired health-related QOL was 5.5 times greater than a healthy child or adolescent and similar to a child or adolescent diagnosed as having cancer."

In adults, the likelihood of patients with impaired glucose tolerance or impaired fasting glucose progressing to diabetes is 25% over 3 to 5 years.[20] There are no large longitudinal studies on children with such data, but smaller studies on at risk populations suggest that there is a high likelihood of progression to type 2 diabetes.[21] Considering the current epidemic of obesity, it is surprising that recent data by the SEARCH for Diabetes in Youth study indicated a low overall prevalence of type 2 diabetes in children.[22] The study found that the overall prevalence of type 1 diabetes was much higher than the prevalence of type 2, with a 1.54 versus 0.22 prevalence per 1000 persons, respectively. However, there were significant ethnic variations when looking at children aged 10 to 19 years. Type 2 diabetes was only 6% of all diabetic cases diagnosed in non-Hispanic whites compared with 22% of all diabetic cases diagnosed in Hispanics. In American Indians, type 2 diabetes has overtaken type 1 in prevalence among children, a startling 72% of all cases of diabetes. The authors suggest that an underestimation of type 2 diabetes may exist considering the difficulties of accurate classification and prompt diagnosis, which is of particular relevance since the SEARCH data were obtained largely through chart review. If rates of obesity continue to rise, while US demographics are growing ethnically diverse, escalating rates of type 2 diabetes in childhood may become an increasing public health concern.

THE DEFINITION OF CHILDHOOD OBESITY AND CONTRIBUTING FACTORS

Targeting childhood obesity is challenging as the very definition of obesity in childhood is controversial. Unlike the definition in adults that relies solely on absolute BMI, the growth curve needs to be taken into account in children. The 2000 growth chart developed by the Centers for Disease Control and Prevention (CDC) is based on national height and weight data for children aged 2 to 19 years. Growth and height are therefore comparative to the reference population, and as charts are revised in the future, they may reflect an overall heavier population. In addition, the CDC and National Heart, Lung and Blood Institute have defined obesity in children as a BMI at or greater than 95% on the 2000 growth chart and overweight as greater than or at 85%. These definitions are arbitrary, and unlike the adult definitions of obesity and overweight, they are not based on health risk data.

The prevention of childhood obesity must take into account factors that have contributed to the growing epidemic of obesity in children. Many of these factors may be similar to those that have contributed to the adult obesogenic environment, including the popularity of fast food, increased transportation by car, and the impact of television (TV) on leisure time. However, there may also be different factors that have contributed to the pediatric obesogenic environment specific to how children spend their time. These factors include how children play, what they do in school, and even changes in how and when they eat. But, similar to adult obesity, ultimately it is the equation of energy balance that becomes lopsided, with increased intake and decreased energy expenditure.

The importance of diet cannot be emphasized enough, but this review focuses on exercise in the prevention of childhood obesity and diabetes. In actuality, most obesity and diabetes prevention trials use a combination of exercise and dietary interventions, as it is necessary to account for both parts of the energy equation to yield meaningful results. Although it is commonly perceived that the culprits of the obesity epidemic are increased time spent by children watching TV and increased fast food intake with larger portion sizes, objective data are difficult to collect on what is likely a multifactorial cause. Social trend data would assist in determining which factors are likely to contribute to obesity, although not necessarily establishing a causal relationship. They would also assist in creating practical interventions to halt the current obesity epidemic.

Specific data are somewhat limited concerning these broad social trends. Survey data in 1997 data compared with those in 1981 indicated that children's free time overall decreased, with increased time spent outside the home, including at school and at day care.[23] Children spent less time eating meals as a primary activity, with more snacking and eating as a secondary activity. Surprisingly some of the survey data indicated that children spent less time watching TV largely due to less leisure time. There was more time spent in structured activities, especially for children younger than 9 years of age, resulting in less unstructured playtime. In terms of other media usage, TV remained the dominant medium overall, but in some groups, other trends emerged. For example, boys aged 8 to 13 years averaged 47 min/d playing video games. The survey data unfortunately did not account for how time was spent in school or at daycare, leaving large gaps in our knowledge base. However, it emphasized that children were spending increasingly longer amounts of time away from home in general. Another study examined transportation to school and found that physically active transportation (ie, walking or biking) to school fell significantly between 1969 and 2001, largely being replaced by automobile transportation to school (Fig. 8).[24] However, the largest decline occurred between 1969 and 1983. Possible reasons for the decline cited by parents included increasing school distance, traffic, sidewalk coverage, fears of "stranger danger," and convenience.

According to CDC data on youth risk behavior for 2005, 21.1% of students used a computer for something that was not schoolwork for 3 or more hours on an average school day.[25] An even greater number of students watched TV, with 37.2% watching

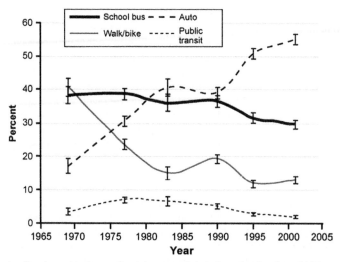

Fig. 8. Standardized mode shares for trips to school. Standardized to 2001 age and race distribution. Error bars represent the 95% confidence intervals. (*From* McDonald NC. Active transportation to school: trends among U.S. schoolchildren, 1969–2001. Am J Prev Med 2007 Jun;32(6):509–16; with permission.)

TV for 3 or more hours per day. In terms of attending gym class, only 54% went to gym class 1 or more days in an average week, and of those who went to gym class, only 84% actually exercised for longer than 20 minutes.

Some studies have focused on finding a direct relationship between factors in the environment and obesity. A randomized, controlled clinical trial found that reducing TV and computer use by 50% in the intervention arm reduced energy intake significantly compared with that in the control group, although there were no significant changes in age- and sex-standardized BMI or physical activity.[26] A cross-sectional study in 2004 including 878 adolescents in the Patient Centered Assessment and Counseling for Exercise Plus Nutrition Project or PACE program studied 7 dietary and physical activity variables and found vigorous physical activity of 60 minutes daily to be the only variable with an independent association with weight status for boys and girls.[27] Physical activity was assessed through the use of accelerometers. One major limitation was that dietary intake was assessed through 24-hour recall, and total calorie intake was actually lower in the overweight group, suggesting that there may have been underreporting in this group compared with normal weight adolescents.

DIABETES OR INSULIN RESISTANCE PREVENTION IN CHILDREN

Unfortunately, there have not been large randomized, controlled trials comparable to the DPP or Finish Diabetes Study for diabetes prevention in children, considering the low incidence of type 2 diabetes in children. To examine such a primary endpoint, long-term follow-up into adulthood would likely be required. However, numerous smaller, randomized, controlled studies have addressed insulin resistance and inflammatory markers in children. There have been many more randomized, controlled trials addressing obesity prevention in children than in adults, as this has been a public health concern that some with foresight had anticipated as far back as 1979 (please refer to appendix 1 for overview studies).[28]

Several small, randomized, controlled trials have looked at metabolic parameters, including insulin sensitivity, cardiovascular fitness as measured by maximum oxygen consumption (VO_2 max), and body composition through either school-based or family-based trials. A randomized, controlled trial on largely first- or second-generation Dominican schoolchildren in New York studied 73 eighth graders who were randomized to either an intervention group that included diet and exercise sessions or the control for 3 to 4 months.[29] The intervention group received on average 14 sessions on nutrition focusing on lower fat intake, and students were given the option of dance or kickboxing classes 3 times a week instead of gym class. About 20 out of the 29 students in the intervention group elected to attend the exercise classes as opposed to regular gym class.

The authors found that CRP was significantly lower in the intervention group compared with that in the control group at the completion of the study. Following the intervention, the percentage of body fat, as measured by bioimpedance, BMI, and IL-6, was significantly lower in the intervention group compared with that in baseline testing. Notably, for both inflammatory markers, CRP and IL-6 differences were only significant for those in the intervention group that participated in both the nutrition sessions and the exercise classes. The quantitative insulin sensitivity check index, or QUICKI score, was higher compared with that in baseline testing in the intervention group, indicating increased insulin sensitivity. The control group did not show any significant changes from baseline testing. There was no significant difference between the groups or from baseline testing in the other factors studied, including lipid profiles, glucose, insulin levels, TNF-α, adipocyte complement-related protein of 30 kDa (adiponectin), and acute insulin response. Actual dietary intake and exercise measurements were not measured (particularly outside of the school setting) and may be confounding variables. Percentage body fat as measured by bioimpedance is affected by hydration state and is not as reliable as other standards such as DXA. However, the study did propose possible changes in physical education curriculum that may be more effective in improving insulin sensitivity compared with traditional gym classes.

Another randomized, controlled study similarly focused on lifestyle-oriented exercise classes compared with standard gym classes.[30] However, this study targeted only children who were already obese with a BMI above the 95% for age. This population was from a rural Wisconsin school compared with inner city students in the Rosenbaum study. The subjects who were randomized to the intervention received educational handouts and were placed in fitness classes of 45 minutes each, with 5 sessions every 2 weeks. These classes encouraged noncompetitive activities, such as walking and cycling, and had only 12 to 14 children per class. The classes increased movement time (42 minutes out of 45) by not having the children change clothes. By contrast, those subjects randomized to the control group participated in traditional gym class, with only 25 minutes of movement time and classes of 35 to 40 students.

The intervention group had significant improvements in VO_2max compared with initial testing ($P<.001$) and with the control group. The intervention group also had significant decreases in both percentage body fat, as measured by DXA, and fasting insulin levels compared with those in initial testing. The intervention group had a significant rise in glucose-insulin ratios compared with baseline testing. There were no significant differences in BMI and fasting glucose level in the intervention group compared with those at baseline testing or control. There were no significant differences in the control group for all variables compared with baseline testing.

This study offered more specific changes that may be instituted in a physical education curriculum, with the goal of improving insulin sensitivity and cardiovascular fitness while decreasing body fat percentage. Although there was no decrease in BMI, other markers of physical fitness improved, emphasizing the benefits of increased exercise. Further studies are needed to evaluate the cost benefit for smaller gym classes, but other formats that increase active time (for example, not changing clothes) are easily implementable. In contrast to the Rosenbaum study, this study targeted obese children only. Although this may be financially more viable, the authors do not comment on any feelings of stigmatization the obese students may have felt toward being separated from their peers. Perhaps it is reassuring that 50 of the 55 students initially invited at the single school enrolled in the study, and only 3 students (5%) dropped out after randomization. However, for public implementation of similar programs this factor is important to consider and address.

Another study, Bright Bodies, also targeted obese students who were above a BMI percentile of 95% on the 2000 CDC chart.[31] Like the Rosenbaum study, this study targeted inner city youth but was family-based rather than school based. The study randomized 209 subjects aged 8 to 16 years in a 2:1 ratio to the intervention and control groups, with an initial further 1:1 randomization in the intervention group to meal structured versus better choices. The meal structured group was dissolved after a high dropout rate (83% of the 35 subjects), and these data were not included in the analysis. The intervention group exercised 50 minutes twice a week at a minimum, with nutrition or behavior classes for 40 minutes once a week for the first 6 months. These were attended by both the parents/caregivers and the children. The exercise classes varied but were high-intensity, including dance, basketball, and sports drills. Subjects wore heart rate (HR) monitors and were encouraged to reach 65% to 85% maximum HR. They were also encouraged to exercise 3 additional days at home per week. During the last 6 months of the study, exercise classes were decreased to twice per month. The control group received diet and exercise counseling twice during the study, at baseline and again at 6 months. The primary endpoint was a change in BMI at 6 months.

The intervention group had decreased BMI and percentage body fat as measured by DXA compared with baseline at 6 months and at 12 months, in contrast to the control group who had an increase in BMI and percentage body fat. Compared with controls, the intervention group also had a decrease in insulin resistance as measured by HOMA-IR scores (Homeostasis Model Assessment of Insulin Resistance— computed by adding fasting insulin and fasting glucose levels and dividing by 22.5). There was a remarkable contrast between the control group whose BMI increased by 1.6 kg/m^2 (a net gain of 7.7 kg) and the intervention group whose BMI declined by 1.7 kg/m^2 (net gain of only 0.3 kg accounted for by an increase in height) during the 12-month period. The study had a high dropout rate even after excluding the arm that was dissolved, with only 119 of the 209 participants completing the study after 12 months. This high dropout rate after enrollment may have introduced some bias. Interestingly, the dropout rates were higher in the control group than those in the Bright Bodies group, which suggests that the intervention introduced practical methods for the subjects to increase activity. However, even with the significant dropout rate, the study was large enough to be adequately powered. In addition, the family-based approach likely yielded some benefits to the caregivers as well, although this was not studied.

Several smaller studies supported these results. One study looked at 15 obese adolescents (BMI >30 kg/m^2) who were randomized to control or intervention for 3 months.[32] The intervention group had weekly nutrition sessions and 45-minute aerobic activity sessions 3 times a week (with 1 session per week monitored, with subjects' parents also participating). The exercise target was gradually achieved in the first 2 weeks. The nutrition sessions focused on low-fat meals, portion control, and limiting soda intake. The intervention group was also encouraged to limit TV use. The control group gained weight, with an increased BMI and body fat percentage measured by DXA during the 3 months, whereas the intervention group maintained weight and BMI. The intervention group had a decreased body fat percentage. In addition, HOMA-IR, CRP, fibrinogen, and IL-6 were decreased in the intervention group compared with those at baseline. There were no significant differences in low-density lipoprotein (LDL), HDL, or triglycerides (TG). This study was quite small with only 7 subjects in the control arm and 8 in the intervention, but it supported the conclusion that increased physical activity improves insulin sensitivity in children.

The second was a Korean study that evaluated 44 obese girls with a BMI >95% based on the Korean Pediatric Association 1998 growth charts. Subjects were randomized to control or lifestyle plus exercise for 12 weeks.[33] The intervention group had supervised sessions of walking 10 minutes on Monday, Wednesday, and Friday and 40 minutes of walking on Tuesday, Thursday, and Saturday. The targeted intensity was 55% to 75% of maximum HR, and the girls wore heart monitors as well as pedometers. The lifestyle intervention included weekly behavior modification sessions with a trained counselor. Subjects kept dietary records in the control and intervention groups, but no significant differences were noted in total caloric intake or macronutrient content. The intervention group had a greater reduction in body weight, BMI, waist circumference, waist-to-hip ratio, systolic blood pressure (SBP), LDL, total cholesterol, glucose, insulin, TG, CRP, leptin, and HOMA-IR. No significant differences were observed in diastolic blood pressure (DBP), HDL, HbA$_{1c}$, or adiponectin compared with those at baseline. This study showed increased insulin sensitivity in obese subjects after an exercise intervention in a population that is increasingly at risk, considering that Asian populations develop diabetes at a higher rate at the same BMI as that of Caucasian populations, with increased propensity for abdominal obesity.

These trials have looked at methods to increase insulin sensitivity, which may delay or prevent the onset of diabetes. The Rosenbaum study was also useful in examining the prevention of obesity by focusing on a general population of children. The other trials mainly had outcomes that could be applied to obesity treatment but not directly to obesity prevention, which is a more immediate and growing public health concern.

FAMILY-BASED OBESITY-PREVENTION TRIALS IN CHILDREN

Several questions arise while formulating obesity-prevention trials. For example, play has always been an essential component of childhood. Even when observing the animal kingdom, we see that young animals' play often models adult behavior. This was likely also true for humans in the premodern era, with children "playing" to fish and hunt while actually learning these skill sets. Children often follow the behaviors of other adults in the community, parents, or caregivers. In the modern world, if children see parents or caregivers using computers frequently even at a young age they desire to imitate them with toy laptops. It is highly likely that sedentary play may lead to decreased physical activity patterns in adulthood. Family-based approaches, where children spend time with parents, increasing physical activity and fitness together, may be more likely to succeed. Even in school-based approaches, without family involvement, the child may feel isolated or be challenged to maintain lifestyle changes in an obesogenic home environment. This possibility has not been addressed in many school-based studies, because activity is often not objectively measured outside the school environment.

Most obesity-prevention trials have been school based, as these are easier to design and implement. However, some family-based trials for obesity prevention have attempted to show that this is another effective approach. A Colorado-based trial focused on a simplified intervention (encouraging an increase in steps per day and cereal consumption) as part of a larger initiative termed America on the Move.[34] The study randomized families who had at least 1 overweight, 8- to 12-year-old child, with a BMI greater than or equal to 85% for age, to control (n = 23) or intervention (n = 82). The intervention group was encouraged to increase steps per day from baseline data to a goal of an additional 2000 steps per day as measured by a pedometer and to eat 2 servings of cereal a day for the 14-week intervention period. The control group also wore pedometers, but the display was turned off, thus not offering feedback. The intervention group increased cereal consumption compared with control but was unable to reach the target of 2 servings per day. In self-reported dietary data, there was no difference in macronutrient intake or total calorie intake between the groups as a result of the intervention.

There was a significant increase in steps approaching an additional 2000 steps in the intervention group compared with that in the control group. There was a decrease in BMI and percentage body fat in the intervention group compared with that in the control. However, when this was analyzed based on sex-specific data, significant decreases in BMI and percentage body fat, as measured by multiple-site, skinfold thickness, were evident only in the girls in the intervention group and not in the boys. Interestingly, this sex-specific difference was also present in the parents, with mothers in the intervention group having significantly decreased BMI and percentage body fat compared with control. The fathers demonstrated a significant difference from baseline (although not control) in change in percentage body fat, which was not evident in the boys.

These sex-specific differences are likely attributable to the design of the study. There was a much larger intervention group (n = 82) than control group (n = 23), which may have caused the study to be underpowered, in particular failing to show a significant difference in the boys (only 8, or 73%, of the control boys completed the study compared with 12, or 86%, of the control girls finishing the study). Because of the small size of the study group, the results of a subgroup analysis may not be valid. Another possibility is that since the boys in the intervention group had an increased number of steps compared with those in the control group, the measurement of percentage body fat by skinfold thickness as a follow-up measure may not be as accurate in young boys as in other populations. The use of skinfold thickness itself lacks the accuracy of other methods in measuring percentage body fat, especially following exercise interventions. A method such as DXA would be preferable, albeit more expensive. Although the study was limited, it demonstrated that children, particularly preadolescents, are capable of increasing their activity levels without specific structured activities. This is especially true with family support and participation. It allows the flexibility for families to pursue activities they enjoy without a regimented approach, leading to an increase in physical fitness.

Another similar family-based study also used pedometers to encourage physical activity but with an open-loop feedback system.[35] Open-loop feedback as opposed to closed-loop feedback involves the participation of a human being, in this case, most likely a parent or other family member, to reinforce certain behaviors. This study randomized children aged 8 to 12 years with a BMI less than 90%, who watched TV or played video games for 15 hours or more per week, to either an open-loop feedback plus reinforcement group or a control group for 6 weeks. The intervention group was encouraged to be physically active and was given TV/video game time based on their activity levels, which was measured by pedometers. About 400 activity units (walking for about 1 hour at 3 mph) were equal to 60 minutes of TV/video game time. Television access was controlled by the caregiver, based on allowance from physical activity units. As in the Colorado study, the control group also wore pedometers but with the display turned off. In this study, the control group was also encouraged in a weekly counseling group to have moderate to vigorous activity for 60 minutes daily. There was no change in BMI z-scores (standard deviations from values that are 50% for sex and age) between the intervention and control groups in the 6-week period of the study. However, physical activity in the intervention group increased by 24% compared with baseline and 32% compared with control, a significant difference. Although the study did not show significant changes in BMI during a relatively short intervention period, it did show increased activity levels that may contribute to obesity prevention in the long-term.

These obesity-prevention trials have attempted to increase unstructured active playtime, because some social trend data have suggested that unstructured playtime has decreased in the past 30 years, especially for younger children. Yet unstructured playtime, to be meaningful, may require space, good weather, safety, and play companions. For example, the 2 family-based studies discussed previously[34,35] were conducted in Colorado and Buffalo, NY, respectively. It is a distinct possibility that the steps taken daily may vary seasonally, with probably less steps being taken during winter as opposed to summer. Additionally, learning structured skill sets may be valuable, as these can be carried on through puberty into adulthood, resulting in a continuum. We speculate that both unstructured and structured playtimes are equally important, with the use of pedometers and open-loop systems being used in younger children and structured activities or sports playing a larger role in older children.

SCHOOL-BASED OBESITY-PREVENTION TRIALS IN CHILDREN

In contrast to these limited family-based trials, a much larger number of trials have been designed as school based. The reason for this becomes evident in that schools offer an easily accessible system already in place for instituting programs. Indeed, other models of school-based interventions, such as smoking cessation, have had considerable success. However, school-based programs also face drawbacks, such as lack of continuity during summer break, the stigmatization of singling out from peers in programs that target only overweight individuals, and the possible lack of family support or knowledge.

As mentioned in the earlier chapter, the Planet Health study randomized schools with a total of 1295 children participating in grades 6 to 7 to either intervention or control for a period of 21 months.[36] The intervention schools taught 16 core lessons focused on 4 behavior modifications, including decreasing TV time, increasing fruit and vegetable consumption to greater than 5 servings per day, decreasing fat intake, and increasing physical activity. The intervention was largely educational with no specific instructions for physical activity. Physical activity and dietary intake were measured through survey data. The intervention group had significant decreases in obesity prevalence (as measured by BMI percentile and triceps skinfold thickness) compared with those in control schools. However, in boys there was no difference between the intervention and control groups. In terms of secondary endpoints, both boys and girls reported a decrease in TV viewing time. The girls in the intervention group also reported a significant decrease in energy intake and an increase in fruit and vegetable consumption compared with those in controls. The study was limited by self-reported data that may have been subject to over- and underreporting. Interestingly, the study found sex-specific differences favoring girls as opposed to boys similar to the Rodearmel study. However, this study was much larger with control and intervention numbers relatively equal (intervention n = 641 and control n = 654). The study suggested that girls are more likely to decrease their dietary intake in response to a behavioral approach. This may be influenced by media emphasis on thinness and dieting, particularly in teenage girls. Although the authors noted that there was no evidence for increases in extreme dieting behaviors among the girls, many adolescents with eating disorders mask their behaviors. Further studies would need to be performed to address these concerns. The Planet Health Study indicated that behavior modification programs may be a useful tool in obesity prevention by decreasing dietary intake. Physical activity did not change between the intervention and control groups based on survey data. A more directed and activity-oriented approach may be required for initiating exercise.

Another large, randomized, controlled trial was conducted in American Indian school children,[37] a high-risk population not only for obesity but for progression to type 2 diabetes of childhood as indicated by SEARCH data. The study randomized 1704 children from third through fifth grade to a Pathways intervention or control for 3 years. The Pathways intervention included weekly nutrition lessons and dietary advice provided to school cafeterias for meal planning. It also included take-home information as well as events for families to attend to bolster family involvement. In terms of physical activity, the Pathways intervention had a minimum of 3 30-minute physical education classes per week with moderate to vigorous activity based on the SPARK program and additional exercise breaks during class for 2 to 10 minutes. There was no change in BMI percentile, % body fat, as measured by bioimpedance, or triceps and subscapular skinfold thickness between the groups. A 24-hour recall showed a significantly lower total and percentage of fat intake in the intervention group. Physical activity as measured by random 24-hour sampling of 15 students in second grade (at baseline) and again at fifth grade showed no difference between the 2 groups.

Interestingly, random sampling accelerometer data did not match with self-reported data, which indicated increased physical activity. Children may have been overreporting activity levels. As seen in overweight adults, overweight children may also underreport intake and may have been more tempted to do so after an intervention emphasizing the importance of healthy eating. One explanation for why the study failed to detect a significant difference in endpoints could be that bioimpedance and skinfold thickness lack adequate accuracy to determine differences in body fat percentages in growing children. An alternative explanation may be that the school did not offer 60 minutes of moderate to vigorous activity per day as suggested by the PACE study. In practical terms, this may be difficult to achieve entirely during school while balancing time for other academic requirements. That the children did not change their physical activity outside of school was likely a confining factor. In addition, there may be ethnic differences in this study population that limit generalizability. The study did not address any change in insulin sensitivity the children may have had, but this may have been a more important and immediate endpoint in this group at high-risk for the development of type 2 diabetes.

Several other large-scale, randomized, controlled trials failed to show a difference between intervention and control groups in the prevention of obesity. A British study performed in Leeds randomized 10 schools to intervention in the active programme promoting lifestyle education in schools (APPLES) program or control for 1 year.[38] The APPLES program was a behavioral modification program, which was designed to target the entire school community, including parents, teachers, and catering staff. It was based on school action plans developed by the individual schools on the basis of their perceived needs. The study had 636 children aged 7 to 11 years and showed no change in BMI or levels of physical activity as measured by questionnaire. There was, however, a significant increase in vegetable consumption based on 24-hour recall in the intervention group compared with that in the control. However, it is unclear in the study how much the intervention differed between the schools in the intervention arm. In addition, there was no direct implementation of increased physical activity during school as far as can be assessed by published data.

Another behavioral study, the Wise Mind Project randomized schools to either a Healthy Eating and Exercise or to a Alcohol/Drug/Tobacco abuse prevention program.[39] The intervention was mainly educational, although teachers were provided with Physical Activity Centers with balls, boanbags, jump ropes, and balloons to encourage indoor and outdoor play during recess. The study had 670 subjects in second to sixth grade and showed no significant differences between the groups in the primary endpoint, z-BMI. There were also no significant changes in secondary endpoints, including body fat percentage as measured by bioimpedance, physical activity as measured by questionnaire, or total calorie intake as measured by digital photography of food leftover on meal plates. The authors suggest that the study was underpowered and thus unable to detect a difference. However, the study did show significant differences in psychosocial variables, another secondary endpoint. The interventional arm had greater self-esteem, less depression, and fewer eating disorder symptoms at the completion of the study compared with those in control as measured by questionnaire.

Another large population-based study adopted an environmental approach rather than a mostly educational one. This study randomized schools with mean enrollments of 1109 students in grades sixth through eighth to an intervention, Middle School Physical Activity and Nutrition program, (M-SPAN), or control for a period of 2 years.[40] The intervention included daily physical education classes and encouraged increased physical activity outside of class as well. Nutritional changes were made in school cafeterias to offer more low-fat choices. In addition, a main component of the program was instituting policy change, which was initiated through health policy meetings and student health committees. There was parental education through newsletters and parent-teacher association meetings and school incentives to participate. Data were collected on food intake and physical activity through direct observation on a random sample. Survey data were collected for out-of school information.

The study found greater physical activity as observed in school in boys in the intervention group compared with that in control but no significant differences in girls. This was also true for out-of school activity. There were no significant differences in total fat intake or saturated fat intake. Unfortunately, BMI was not measured in this study but was self-reported. BMI declined for boys and not for the girls according to self-reported data. Interestingly, this study also found sex-specific differences but the opposite of those found in Planet Health. The possible reasons for this may have been increased self-consciousness by girls during observation while exercising. It is unclear if the physical education classes in this study were coed, another factor that could have influenced the behavior of both boys as well as girls. The study was significantly limited by not gathering objective data in terms of BMI. The study did offer a different perspective in creating a school environment that was more conducive to a healthy lifestyle, which may have facilitated increased physical activity, especially for boys. The study attempted to alter the school environment to be less obesogenic, although significant environmental forces outside of school remained unaffected.

Another school-based study took an academic and educational approach, randomizing 1013 fourth and fifth graders to intervention or control.[41] The Wellness, Academics and You, or "WAY" program integrated healthy behaviors into the academic curriculum by teaching 7 modules in subjects as diverse as language, mathematics, and science. The program had 10-minute aerobic exercise routines before the breaks during class in the interventional group. The interventional group had a 2% reduction in overweight (or BMI greater than 85%), but the authors state there were no significant changes in reported physical activity levels or nutritional uptake. There was a trend toward increased activity and increased fruit and vegetable consumption. The study could not determine the actual factors that resulted in the weight loss, but it offered a possible solution for schools in balancing time for academics and physical fitness. In fact, survey data from the teachers indicated improved attention and focus from the students in the interventional arm.

Perhaps these studies indicate that a combination of environmental, behavioral, and educational components is necessary for meaningful results in obesity prevention. Some limitations of many of these studies have been a lack of objective data with regard to actual physical activity performed, perhaps better gathered through accelerometer data, and dietary intake. It is possible that more structured interventions that increase physical activity, such as those performed in the Bright Bodies or Carrell studies, may ease student initiation toward becoming more physically active.

A 3-year randomized, controlled, international study in Beijing, China, in 2007 reported remarkably large decreases in obesity prevalence.[42] The study randomized primary schools (grades 1–4) to intervention or control, with a total of 2425 students. The study was conducted over 3 years. The intervention consisted of nutritional lectures with handouts once per semester for parents and didactic lessons every 2 weeks for the children in school on topics related to obesity prevention. In addition, there were interactive meetings for the parents of overweight or obese children once per semester as well as separate meetings for the overweight children. Mondays through Thursdays, overweight children and those children who failed physical education were asked to run for 20 minutes after class and were monitored. BMI was measured and calculated with age-specific and sex-specific percentiles, as recommended by the International Obesity Taskforce.

At the end of the study, the intervention schools had significantly lower overweight prevalence rates than those in the control schools, a 26.3% decrease compared with 14.3% increase. Obesity prevalence decreased in the intervention arm 32.5% compared with an increase in the control arm of 15.7%. This study showed startling differences in obesity outcome rates in contrast to other studies. Some factors that may have led to increased success rates in this trial may be that it was longer in duration, involved younger children, and involved significant parent participation. In particular, nutritional recommendations concerning meal preparation for the parents may have had a significant effect, perhaps amplified by differences in Chinese dietary habits. The study authors also noted that cultural differences may have contributed to overfeeding in single-child households (as most households are in China), with boys being overweight or obese at higher rates than girls. The study interventional arm specifically addressed this behavior, which may have had a significant effect on decreasing calorie intake. In addition, this study had a dramatically different ethnic composition than the prior American and European studies mentioned, which may have played a significant role.

In an effort to concentrate resources, the Chinese study targeted obese and overweight children, as did many of the other obesity-prevention studies. It is unclear if children felt stigmatized by this separation. In addition, with a rapidly increased percentage of the population at risk for obesity, it may be self-defeating not to address obesity prevention in the general population. One challenge with population-based programs, however, is ensuring safety. Would thin children be at risk for losing weight or having a deceleration in growth? In the study by Jiang and colleagues,[42] children in the intervention group and the control group had similar linear growth velocities. Many of the other trials noted that there were no adverse effects reported as a result of the intervention. The Pathways study identified children below the third percentile in growth velocity and referred them to their primary care provider, but it also noted that this number did not change as a result of the intervention.

As the American environment has grown more obesogenic, media images of what is considered attractive have trended in the opposing direction. This is particularly true in the case of women where advertisements routinely feature females who are under-weight, with a BMI less than 18 kg/m². In this social context, an important question is whether programs designed to prevent diabetes or obesity through increasing phys-ical activity and discussing food choices would place teenage girls or other high-risk populations at risk for eating disorders. This situation is similar to one that has already been encountered in adolescents with type 1 diabetes. A cross-sectional study of 356 girls with type 1 diabetes found a higher prevalence of eating disorders, including bulimia, compared with controls without diabetes.[43] Some reasons for this may be increased weight gain after the initiation of insulin and the intensified focus on food choices necessary for the management of diabetes.

Some of the randomized, controlled trials addressed this concern. Authors of the Wise Mind Study found a decrease in the risk of eating disorder behaviors following the intervention. A school-based study called New Moves tried to minimize self-consciousness for adolescent girls while participating in physical education by offering girls-only classes.[44] Indeed self-consciousness in adolescent girls may be one reason the M-SPAN study observed a decrease in physical activity in girls compared with that in boys during school. A recent study using accelerometer data indicated that moderate to physical activity decreases between the ages of 9 to 15, with girls being less active than boys.[45]

The New Moves Program was advertised as a program to increase physical activity and help with healthy weight management. The intervention group received girls-only classes 4 days a week, which included noncompetitive activities, such as aerobic dance, yoga, and kickboxing, rather than traditional coed gym classes as in the control group. There was also 1 weight training session a week, with a nutrition/social support session every other week. Although the intervention group showed no significant changes in BMI at the end of the study, the program seemed to have a positive impact and was well received by the students.

As children have growing academic demands and greater time spent away from home, an alternative approach may be afterschool programs. The Georgia FitKid project was designed to increase moderate to vigorous physical activity after school.[46] The study randomized schools to either intervention or control, with 601 third graders participating for 1 year. The intervention was for 2 hours after school in which the first 40 minutes were spent assisting children with homework. They received a snack during this period following United States Department of Agriculture USDA guidelines for nutritional content. This was followed by an 80-minute period of exer-cise, which had 40 minutes of moderate to vigorous activity, with games such as tag, basketball, and soccer. About 5% of subjects wore HR monitors during the sessions. There was a significant decrease in percentage of body fat as measured by DXA in the intervention group as compared with the control. In addition, there was a significant improvement in cardiovascular fitness (as assessed by HR in

Appendix 1

Study Name and Type	# of Subjects, Age, Population, and Length of Study	Diet Intervention	Exercise Intervention	Outcome
Rosenbaum et al School-based	73 eighth graders First- or second-generation Dominicans in New York City 3–4 mo	14 nutrition sessions	Dance or kickboxing 3 times a week instead of traditional gym class	↓ CRP intervention vs control ↓ % body fat (BF) by bioimpedance, BMI, and IL-6 intervention group vs baseline testing ↑ QUIKI score intervention vs control No Δ lipid profiles, glucose levels, insulin levels. TNF-α, adiponectin, and acute in sulin response to glucose
Carrel et al School-based	50 obese middle school children Rural Wisconsin School 9 mo	Educational handouts	Smaller fitness classes instead of traditional gym, 5 times in a 2-wk period	↑ VO₂ max intervention vs baseline and contro ↓ % BF by DXA, fasting insulin, glucose-insulin ratios vs baseline No Δ BMI and fasting glucose
Savoye et al "Bright Bodies" Family-based	209 obese children ages 8–16 y Inner city population 6–12 mo	Intervention group—nutrition/behavior classes 40 min/wk for 6 mo and then every other week Control group—diet and exercise counseling twice during the study	High-intensity exercise classes 50 min twice a week at a minimum for 6 mo, then twice per month	↓ BMI percentile, BF % by DXA intervention vs baseline ↓ HOMA-IR intervention vs control ↑ BMI percentile, % BF by DXA control vs baseline
Balogopal et al Family-based	15 obese adolescents 3 mo	Weekly nutrition sessions	45-min aerobic activity sessions 3 times a week (with 1 session per week monitored)	↓ BF % by DXA intervention vs baseline and control ↓ HOMA-IR, CRP, fibrinogen, and IL-6 intervention vs baseline ↑BMI percentile and % BF by DXA control vs baseline No Δ in LDL, HDL, or TG
Park et al School-based	44 obese girls Ages 13–15 y Korean city population 12 wk	Weekly behavior modification sessions with a trained counselor	Supervised sessions of walking 10 min Monday, Wednesday, Friday and 40 min Tuesday, Thursday, Saturday, Sunday	↓ BMI percentile, waist circumference, waist/hip ratio, SBP, LDL, total cholesterol, glucose, insu in, TG, CRP, leptin, and HOMA-IR in intervention vs control No Δ DBP, HDL, HbA₁c or adiponectin

Appendix 2

Study Name and Type	# of Subjects, Ages, Population, and Length of Study	Diet Intervention	Exercise Intervention	Outcome
Rodearmel et al "America on the Move" Family-based	105 families with at least 1 overweight child aged 8–12 y Fort Collins area, Colorado 13 wk	Consumption of 2 servings of cereal a day	increase steps per day from baseline data to a goal of an additional 2000 steps/day as measured by pedometer	↑In steps approaching an additional 2000 steps in intervention group vs control ↓ BMI percentile and % BF by skinfold thickness intervention vs control On further sex-specific analysis ↓BMI and BF % was seen only in girls, not in boys
Roemmich et al "Open-Loop Feedback" Family-based	18 families with children aged 8–12 y with BMI <90% who watched TV/played video games for ≥15 h/wk Buffalo, NY 6 wk	None	Intervention group— TV/video game time given based on activity levels measured by pedometers Control group— weekly counseling group to encourage moderate to vigorous activity for 60 min daily	↑ Physical activity in the intervention group vs baseline and control No Δ in BMI z-scores
Gortmaker et al "Planet Health" School-based	10 schools with 1295 children grades 6–7 Ethnically diverse communities in Massachusetts 21 mo	Lessons emphasizing ↑ fruit and vegetable to >5 servings per day, and ↓fat intake	Lessons emphasizing ↓TV time and ↑physical activity	↓ BMI percentile and BF % by kinfold thickness intervention vs controls Sex-specific analysis showed no difference in boys ↓ TV time based on survey data for boys and girls ↓Energy intake in girls based on survey data intervention vs control ↑Fruit and vegetable consumption in girls based on survey data intervention vs control

Study	Nutrition Intervention	Physical Activity Intervention	Outcomes
Callerbero et al "Pathways" School-based	1704 children third through fifth grades American Indian schools in Arizona, South Dakota, and New Mexico 3 y	Weekly nutrition lessons Dietary advice provided to school cafeterias for meal planning Take-home information and events for families	Minimum of 3 30-min gym classes per week based on the SPARK program Additional exercise breaks during class for 2-10 minutes	No Δ BMI percentile, % BF as measured by bioimpedance or skinfold thickness ↓ Total and percentage of fat intake by a 24-hour recall in intervention vs control
Sahota et al School-based	10 schools with 637 children aged 7-11 y Leeds, England 1 y	A behavioral modification program "APPLES" targeting parents, teachers, and catering staff. Based on school action plans developed by the individual schools	Behavioral modification program "APPLES"	No Δ in BMI, no Δ physical activity as measured by questionnaire ↑ In vegetable consumption based on 24-h recall in the intervention vs control
Williamson et al "Wise Mind Project" School-based	4 private Catholic schools with 670 students in second to sixth grade Louisiana 2 y	Educational program using posters, handouts, displays Wise Mind staff works with cafeteria on improving school lunches	Teachers given physical activity centers to encourage indoor and outdoor play	No Δ z-BMI or BF % by bioimpedance No Δ physical activity as measured by questionnaire or calorie intake as measured by digital photography of food leftover on meal plates
Sallis et al School-based	48 schools with 1109 students grades sixth through eighth San Diego County, CA 2 y	More low-fat choices in school cafeterias	Daily physical education classes Physical activity outside of class encouraged	↑ Physical activity as observed in school in boys in the intervention vs control No Δ in physical activity as observed in girls No Δ in total fat intake or saturated fat intake as observed by random sample observation BMI was not measured

(continued on next page)

Appendix 2
(continued)

Study Name and Type	# of Subjects, Ages, Population, and Length of Study	Diet Intervention	Exercise Intervention	Outcome
Spiegel and Foulk "The WAY program" School-based	1013 fourth and fifth graders Delaware, Florida, Kansas, North Carolina 5–6 mo	Educational module on nutrition	Educational module on designing basic workout routines 10-minute aerobic exercise routines before the breaks during class	↓ Reduction (2%) in overweight intervention vs control No Δ in reported physical activity levels or nutritional uptake
Jiang et al School-based	Primary schools (grades 1–4) with a total of 2425 students Beijing, China 3 y	Nutritional lectures for the parents 1x/semester Lessons and handouts every 2 wk for the children	Run for 20 min after class twice a week	↓ Overweight prevalence rates intervention vs control
Neumark-Sztainer et al "New Moves" School-based	6 schools with 201 girls Twin cities area, Minnesota 16 wk	Nutritional sessions every other week	4 d a week fitness sessions instead of traditional gym class, included weight training weekly, community guest instructors, lifestyle-oriented activities	No Δ BMI
Yin et al "Georgia FitKid Project" Afterschool program	18 schools with 601 third graders Georgia 8 mo (data published) Study ongoing, planned for 3 y	Afterschool snack following USDA guidelines	80 min period of exercise, which had 40 min of moderate to vigorous activity	Using subjects who attended ≥40% sessions—↓BF % by DXA in ↓HR in response to 3-min bench stepping test ↑ bone mineral density in intervention vs control No Δ in BMI, blood pressure, and lipid profiles Using intention to treat analysis no Δ in any of the endpoints

response to 3-minute bench stepping test) and bone mineral density in the intervention group compared with the control. There were no significant differences in BMI, BP, or lipid profiles. However, this was based on data that only included children who attended more than 40% of the sessions (182 out of the initial 312 in the intervention group). When the data were reanalyzed using intention to treat, there was no significant difference. Perhaps this indicates that the method used in the study may have been effective at preventing obesity, but the practicality of afterschool programs is open to questions, particularly when considering barriers to attendance. Some of these may include difficulty with transportation and other conflicting afterschool commitments.

However, the Georgia FitKid program was largely designed to increase activity during a time of day that might have been spent in largely sedentary activities for many kids, such as watching TV after school. Indeed in this age of technology, TV, the Internet, and videogames are increasingly blamed for contributing to the rise in obesity. Yet these increasingly pervasive technologies are difficult to avoid. One possible solution would be to use technology to increase activity. The use of pedometers as useful technological devices in obesity prevention has been demonstrated, as discussed in prior studies. An innovative, randomized, controlled study designed a program that creatively used a videogame, pedometer, and parental involvement to increase activity.[47] The study randomized children aged 9 to 11 years to a futuristic videogame called MetaKenkoh or to control. The game involved accumulating steps on a pedometer, which were then downloaded into the program. The steps permit the child to continue progressing in and playing the videogame. Analysis of preliminary data indicated after 1 week that the intervention group had increased activity compared with baseline, whereas the control group had a drop in steps. Continued interest in the game as well as duration of interest remain to be determined. However, such an approach may be useful in combining active approaches to mainly sedentary activities. This may be likened to the expenditures that occur while playing videogames such as Wii Fit.[48]

SUMMARY AND RECOMMENDATIONS

Most of the randomized, controlled studies addressing prevention of obesity in children do not show a decrease in BMI. Programs that have significant increases in moderate to vigorous physical activity during monitored sessions or as measured by objective data seem to show the greatest benefits. Although they do not often result in a significant decrease in BMI, most trials that use accurate measures have reported a significant decrease in percentage body fat. These trials have also shown improvements in markers of insulin resistance and inflammation through physical activity. The benefits of exercise thus extend beyond weight loss. Exercise alters the distribution of fat by decreasing visceral obesity. In addition, it contributes to increased insulin sensitivity and decreased inflammation. Perhaps focusing on obesity prevention as an endpoint is misguided, and studies should be designed to increase fitness and healthy eating. Focusing on fitness may demonstrate more immediate results and initiate lifestyle changes in subjects. This would embody a positive rather than a negative approach and in the long-term decrease overall rates of obesity.

Consensus Guidelines from 2005 have recommended that schools have 30 to 34 minutes of strenuous activity daily and that, in general, sedentary activity should be restricted.[49] In 2008, published guidelines from the Endocrine Society have recommended that clinicians recommend 60 minutes of daily moderate to vigorous physical activity for children.[50] In addition, they also recommend limiting screen time to 1 to 2 hours daily. Although citing several studies to support these recommendations, both guidelines concur that there are limited quality data provided by obesity-prevention studies. However, they also state that lack of conclusive data should not preclude action toward obesity prevention.

One conundrum in designing randomized, controlled trials for the prevention of obesity and its associated complications is the issue of achieving a balance between an adequately powered study and one that also has accuracy. To have statistical significance and be adequately powered as well as to be considered a true population study, a large number of subjects are required. However, this often results in poorer measures of outcomes, with less objective data collected. Often studies will rely on survey data rather than direct measurement of physical activity, such as the use of an accelerometer, because they are less expensive and time consuming. Similarly, measurements of body fat percentage in many large trials have relied on skinfold thickness or bioimpedance, which is less accurate than DXA. Another barrier has been the significant duration of time needed to show treatment differences, especially in reduction of BMI.

Finally, rather than focusing on 1 type of intervention, multiple interventions are needed depending on the age, environment, and risk factors for the child. Younger children may benefit from more unstructured play and adolescents may benefit from programs that offer activities that will be available in the community as they transition to adulthood. School-based interventions could be implemented together with family-based involvement, such as evening sessions or parental monitoring of accelerometer usage. Resources could be allocated to design high-intensity interventions, such as the Bright Bodies program, to address populations most at risk for the complications of obesity, such as the American Indian population. Further funding could be broadly distributed in low-cost interventions to revise existing physical education programs. Some low-cost interventions might include increasing actual activity time, perhaps by separating girls and boys or by not having children change clothes.

Interventions to increase exercise should lay the foundations for a healthy lifestyle that can be maintained throughout adulthood. This will, in turn, result in healthier pregnancies, parenting, and in turn teach the next generation these same behaviors.

REFERENCES

1. Kung HC, Hoyert DL, Xu JQ, et al. Deaths: final data for 2005. National vital statistics reports, vol. 56 No 10. Hyattsville (MD): National Center for Health Statistics; 2008.
2. Ogden CL, Carroll MD, McDowell MA, et al. Obesity among adults in the United States- no change since 2003–2004. NCHS data brief no 1. Hyattsville (MD): National Center for Health Statistics; 2007.
3. Ogden CL, Carroll MD, Flegal KM. High body mass index for age among US children and adolescents, 2003–2006. JAMA 2008;299(20):2401–5.
4. Kelly T, Yang W, Chen CS, et al. Global burden of obesity in 2005 and projections to 2030. Int J Obes (Lond) 2008;32(9):1431–7.
5. de Onis M, Blössner M. Prevalence and trends of overweight among preschool children in developing countries. Am J Clin Nutr 2000;72(4):1032–9.
6. Eiben G, Lissner L. Health hunters–an intervention to prevent overweight and obesity in young high-risk women. Int J Obes (Lond) 2006;30(4):691–6.

7. Irwin ML, Yasui Y, Ulrich CM, et al. Effect of exercise on total and intra-abdominal body fat in postmenopausal women: a randomized controlled trial. JAMA 2003; 289(3):323–30.

8. Tuomilehto J, Lindstrom J, Eriksson JG, et al. Prevention of type 2 diabetes mellitus by changes in lifestyle among subjects with impaired glucose tolerance. N Engl J Med 2001;344:1343–50.

9. Lindström J, Ilanne-Parikka P, Peltonen M, et al. Sustained reduction in the incidence of type 2 diabetes by lifestyle intervention: follow-up of the Finnish Diabetes Prevention Study. Lancet 2006;368(9548):1673–9.

10. Saaristo T, Peltonen M, Keinänen-Kiukaanniemi S, et al. National type 2 diabetes prevention programme in Finland: FIN-D2D. Int J Circumpolar Health 2007;66(2): 101–12.

11. Knowler WC, Barrett-Connor E, Fowler SE, et al. Reduction in the incidence of type 2 diabetes with lifestyle intervention or metformin. N Engl J Med 2002;346: 393–403.

12. Knowler WC, Barrett-Connor E, Fowler SE, et al. Effects of withdrawal from metformin on the development of diabetes in the diabetes prevention program. Diabetes Care 2003;26(4):977–80. Comment on: Diabetes Care. 2003 Apr;26(4): 1306–8.

13. Li G, Zhang P, Wang J, et al. The long-term effect of lifestyle interventions to prevent diabetes in the China Da Qing Diabetes Prevention Study: a 20-year follow-up study. Lancet 2008;371(9626):1783–9.

14. Pan XR, Li GW, Hu YH, et al. Effects of diet and exercise in preventing NIDDM in people with impaired glucose tolerance. The Da Qing IGT and Diabetes Study. Diabetes Care 1997;20:37–44.

15. Wadden TA, Crerand CE, Brock J. Behavioral treatment of obesity. Psychiatr Clin North Am 2005;28(1):151–70.

16. Pietrobelli A, Malavolti M, Battistini NC, et al. Metabolic syndrome: a child is not a small adult. Int J Pediatr Obes 2008;3(Suppl 1):67–71.

17. Magarey AM, Daniels LA, Boulton TJ, et al. Predicting obesity in early adulthood from childhood and parental obesity. Int J Obes Relat Metab Disord 2003;27(4): 505–13.

18. Weiss R, Dziura J, Burgert TS, et al. Obesity and the metabolic syndrome in children and adolescents. N Engl J Med 2004;350(23):2362–74.

19. Schwimmer JB, Burwinkle TM, Varni JW. Health-related quality of life of severely obese children and adolescents. JAMA 2003;289(14):1813–9.

20. Nathan DM, Davidson MB, DeFronzo A, et al. Impaired fasting glucose and impaired glucose tolerance: implications for care. Diabetes Care 2007;30:753–9.

21. Weiss R, Taksali SE, Tamborlane WV, et al. Predictors of changes in glucose tolerance status in obese youth. Diabetes Care 2005;28:902–9.

22. Liese AD, D'Agostino RB Jr, Hamman RF, et al. The burden of diabetes mellitus among US youth: prevalence estimates from the SEARCH for Diabetes in Youth Study. SEARCH for Diabetes in Youth Study Group. Pediatrics 2006;118(4): 1510–8.

23. Hofferth SL, Sandberg JF. Changes in American children's time, 1981–1997. Children at the millennium: where have we come from, where are we going? Advances in life course research. New York: Elsevier Science; 2001.

24. McDonald NC. Active transportation to school: trends among U.S. schoolchildren, 1969–2001. Am J Prev Med 2007;32(6):509–16.

25. Eaton DK, Kann L, Kinchen S, et al. Youth risk behavior surveillance–United States, 2005. MMWR Surveill Summ 2006;55(5):1–108.

26. Epstein LH, Roemmich JN, Robinson JL, et al. A randomized trial of the effects of reducing television viewing and computer use on body mass index in young children. Arch Pediatr Adolesc Med 2008;162(3):239–45.
27. Patrick K, Norman GJ, Calfas KJ, et al. Diet, physical activity, and sedentary behaviors as risk factors for overweight in adolescence. Arch Pediatr Adolesc Med 2004;158(4):385–90.
28. Botvin GJ, Cantlon A, Carter BJ, et al. Reducing adolescent obesity through a school health program. J Pediatr 1979;95(6):1060–3.
29. Rosenbaum M, Nonas C, Weil R, et al. School-based intervention acutely improves insulin sensitivity and decreases inflammatory markers and body fatness in junior high school students. J Clin Endocrinol Metab 2007;92(2):504–8.
30. Carrel AL, Clark RR, Peterson SE, et al. Improvement of fitness, body composition, and insulin sensitivity in overweight children in a school-based exercise program: a randomized, controlled study. Arch Pediatr Adolesc Med 2005; 159(10):963–8.
31. Savoye M, Shaw M, Dziura J, et al. Effects of a weight management program on body composition and metabolic parameters in overweight children: a randomized controlled trial. JAMA 2007;297(24):2697–704.
32. Balagopal P, George D, Patton N, et al. Lifestyle-only intervention attenuates the inflammatory state associated with obesity: a randomized controlled study in adolescents. J Pediatr 2005;146(3):342–8.
33. Park TG, Hong HR, Lee J, et al. Lifestyle plus exercise intervention improves metabolic syndrome markers without change in adiponectin in obese girls. Ann Nutr Metab 2007;51(3):197–203.
34. Rodearmel SJ, Wyatt HR, Barry MJ, et al. A family-based approach to preventing excessive weight gain. Obesity (Silver Spring) 2006;14(8):1392–401.
35. Roemmich JN, Gurgol CM, Epstein LH. Open-loop feedback increases physical activity of youth. Med Sci Sports Exerc 2004;36(4):668–73.
36. Gortmaker SL, Peterson K, Wiecha J, et al. Reducing obesity via a school-based interdisciplinary intervention among youth: Planet Health. Arch Pediatr Adolesc Med 1999;153(4):409–18.
37. Caballero B, Clay T, Davis SM, et al. Pathways: a school-based, randomized controlled trial for the prevention of obesity in American Indian schoolchildren. Am J Clin Nutr 2003;78(5):1030–8.
38. Sahota P, Rudolf MC, Dixey R, et al. Randomised controlled trial of primary school based intervention to reduce risk factors for obesity. BMJ 2001;323(7320): 1029–32.
39. Williamson DA, Copeland AL, Anton SD, et al. Wise Mind project: a school-based environmental approach for preventing weight gain in children. Obesity (Silver Spring) 2007;15(4):906–17.
40. Sallis JF, McKenzie TL, Conway TL, et al. Environmental interventions for eating and physical activity: a randomized controlled trial in middle schools. Am J Prev Med 2003;24(3):209–17.
41. Spiegel SA, Foulk D. Reducing overweight through a multidisciplinary school-based intervention. Obesity (Silver Spring) 2006;14(1):88–96.
42. Jiang J, Xia X, Greiner T, et al. The effects of a 3-year obesity intervention in schoolchildren in Beijing. Child Care Health Dev 2007;33(5):641–6.
43. Jones J, Lawson ML, Daneman D, et al. Eating disorders in adolescent females with and without type I diabetes mellitus: cross-sectional study. BMJ 2000;320: 1563–6.

44. Neumark-Sztainer D, Story M, Hannan PJ, et al. New Moves: a school-based obesity prevention program for adolescent girls. Prev Med 2003;37(1):41–51.
45. Nader PR, Bradley RH, Houts RM, et al. Moderate-to-vigorous physical activity from ages 9 to 15 years. JAMA 2008;300(3):295–305.
46. Yin Z, Gutin B, Johnson MH, et al. An environmental approach to obesity prevention in children: Medical College of Georgia FitKid Project year 1 results. Obes Res 2005;13(12):2153–61.
47. Southard DR, Southard BH. Promoting physical activity in children with MetaKenkoh. Clin Invest Med 2006;29(5):293–7.
48. Graves LE, Ridgers ND, Stratton G. The contribution of upper limb and total body movement to adolescents' energy expenditure whilst playing Nintendo Wii. Eur J Appl Physiol 2008;104(4):617–23.
49. Speiser PW, Rudolf MC, Anhalt H, et al. Childhood obesity. J Clin Endocrinol Metab 2005;90(3):1871–87. Epub 2004 Dec 14. Review.
50. August GP, Caprio S, Fennoy I, et al. Prevention and treatment of pediatric obesity: an endocrine society clinical practice guideline based on expert opinion. J Clin Endocrinol Metab 2009;93(12):4576–99.

The Use of Exercise in the Management of Type 1 and Type 2 Diabetes

Nathan Y. Weltman, Med[a],*, Susan A. Saliba, PhD, PT, ATC[b],
Eugene J. Barrett, MD, PhD[c], Arthur Weltman, PhD, FACSM[d,e]

KEYWORDS

- Prediabetes • Metabolic syndrome • Exercise prescription
- Exercise training • Strength training

Diabetes Mellitus is an illness that requires intensive, daily medical care and patient self-management education to both reduce the risk of acute complications and to improve long-term outcomes. Clinical interventions used to improve the management of diabetes include medical therapy, nutritional therapy, diabetes self-management education, psychosocial assessment and care, hypoglycemia awareness management, immunizations, and exercise.[1] Exercise is also an effective intervention in individuals with a high risk for developing diabetes, that is, individuals with either impaired fasting glucose (IFG) or glucose tolerance and metabolic syndrome. This article first reviews the data supporting the effectiveness of exercise evaluation and prescription programs in promoting cardiovascular health. Subsequently, the use of and restrictions to exercise in improving the management and reducing potential complications from type 1 and type 2 diabetes (T1D and T2D) in children, adolescents, and adults are discussed.

[a] Sanford School of Medicine, University of South Dakota, 414 E Clark Street, Lee Medical Building, Vermillion, SD 57069, USA
[b] Department of Human Services, Curry School of Education, University of Virginia, 210 Emmett Street, Charlottesville, VA 22904, USA
[c] Department of Medicine, School of Medicine, University of Virginia, 210 Emmett Street, Charlottesville, VA 22904, USA
[d] Department of Human Services, Curry School of Education, University of Virginia, 210 Emmett Street, Charlottesville, VA 22904, USA
[e] School of Medicine, University of Virginia, 210 Emmett Street, Charlottesville, VA 22904, USA
* Corresponding author.
E-mail address: nathan.weltman@usd.edu (N.Y. Weltman).

Clin Sports Med 28 (2009) 423–439
doi:10.1016/j.csm.2009.02.006
0278-5919/09/$ – see front matter © 2009 Elsevier Inc. All rights reserved.
sportsmed.theclinics.com

DIABETES CLASSIFICATION
Type 1 Diabetes

Also known as either immune-mediated diabetes, insulin-dependent diabetes, or juvenile onset diabetes, T1D accounts for ~5% to 10% of diabetes in the United States. T1D is caused by autoimmune destruction of β cells of the pancreas and usually leads to absolute insulin deficiency. The rate of β-cell destruction is rapid in infants and children and relatively slower in adults. Individuals present with either severe metabolic decompensation with ketoacidosis or modest, fasting hyperglycemia that can rapidly change to severe hyperglycemia or ketoacidosis in the presence of infection or other stressors. Some individuals with T1D, particularly adults, maintain residual β-cell function for many years. Most of these individuals eventually become insulin dependent.[1,2]

A subset of patients with T1D, primarily African Americans and Asians, develop diabetes and can present with ketoacidosis, yet do not have evidence of autoimmune β-cell destruction. This form of T1D appears to have a hereditary basis, but the pathogenesis is unclear. These individuals may experience episodic, severe metabolic decompensation including ketoacidosis and need intermittent insulin replacement therapy.

Type 2 Diabetes

Approximately 90% to 95% of individuals with diabetes have T2D, also known as either non–insulin-dependent diabetes or adult-onset diabetes. Individuals with T2D have insulin resistance, which ranges from predominantly insulin resistance and relative insulin deficiency to predominantly insulin resistance with an insulin secretory defect.[2] These patients usually do not require insulin treatment early in the course of their disease, but as many as 50% eventually become insulin dependent to maintain metabolic control.

There is a strong genetic predisposition to the development of T2D. It is a polygenic disorder, and although multiple risk alleles have been identified, the complex genetics of this form of diabetes is not well defined.[2] Women with a history of gestational diabetes mellitus (GDM) and individuals with either hypertension or dyslipidemia, or both, are also at increased risk. The risk of developing T2D increases with age, obesity, and sedentary lifestyle. Notably, T2D diagnosis is often delayed for several years, partly because hyperglycemia develops gradually, and the classic symptoms of polyuria and polydipsia are not prominent during the early stages. However, most of these patients have signs of prediabetes or metabolic syndrome, which can be treated by virtually identical exercise management techniques.

Other Types of Diabetes

Other, less common forms of diabetes include autosomal dominant genetic defects in β-cell function and insulin action, diabetes secondary to diseases of the pancreas (eg, pancreatitis), diabetes secondary to endocrine pathology (eg, acromegaly, Cushing's syndrome), drug- or chemical-induced diabetes, uncommon forms of immune-mediated diabetes, genetic syndromes associated with diabetes, and GDM.

GDM refers to any degree of glucose intolerance that is first noted during pregnancy. In the last trimester, insulin resistance progressively increases secondary to changes in body weight and the release of hormones by the placentas, which in turn antagonize insulin action. GDM complicates ~4% of pregnancies in the United States (~135,000 annually).

DIAGNOSIS

The American Diabetes Association (ADA) recommends use of the fasting glucose test to diagnose diabetes in children and nonpregnant, *symptomatic* adults.[1] The current criteria for the diagnosis of diabetes include 1 of the following:

1. Fasting blood glucose greater than or equal to 126 mg/dL (7.0 mmol/L). Fasting is defined as zero-caloric intake for at least 8 hours before the test.[f]
2. Symptoms of hyperglycemia and a *casual* blood glucose greater than or equal to 200 mg/dL (11.1 mmol/L). *Casual* is defined as any time of day without regard to time since the last meal. The classic symptoms of hyperglycemia include polyuria, polydipsia, and unexplained weight loss.
3. Two-hour blood glucose greater than or equal to 200 mg/dL (11.1 mmol/L) during an oral glucose tolerance test (OGTT), using a glucose load containing the equivalent of 75 g anhydrous glucose dissolved in water.[f]

Diagnosis of Prediabetes

Individuals who are hyperglycemic but do not meet the definition of diabetes can be categorized as having prediabetes by either IFG, fasting blood glucose 100 mg/dL (5.6 mmol/L) to 125 mg/dL (6.9 mmol/L), or impaired glucose tolerance (IGT), 2-hour blood glucose 140 mg/dL (7.8 mmol/L) to 199 mg/dL (11.0 mmol/L).[1] Both IFG and IGT are associated with increased risk for the future development of diabetes and increased risk for cardiovascular disease (CVD).[4]

The metabolic syndrome is a prediabetic state that is associated with increased cardiometabolic risk.[5,6] Both the National Cholesterol Education Program (NCEP) Expert Panel on Detection, Evaluation, and Treatment of High Blood Cholesterol in Adults (Adult Treatment Panel III [NCEP-ATP III])[7,8] and the International Diabetes Federation (IDF)[9] criteria use 5 risk factors—waist circumference, triglycerides, blood pressure, HDL cholesterol, and fasting glucose—to determine the presence of metabolic syndrome. The NCEP-ATP III guidelines require the presence of any 3 of 5 risk factors, whereas the IDF criteria require elevated waist circumference, because of the relationship between abdominal obesity and cardiometabolic risk,[9,10] and 2 of the remaining 4 risk factors. However, the 5 risk factors are not used as continuous variables but rather counted as "present" or "absent." Therefore, the efficacy of these screening tools is less than optimal for assigning risk for the metabolic syndrome.[10]

Diagnosis of Diabetes and Prediabetes in Asymptomatic Individuals

Many asymptomatic individuals who wish to engage in exercise programs would benefit from testing to detect prediabetes and diabetes before exercise evaluation. The ADA has developed guidelines for asymptomatic patients who should be considered for testing.[1]

Screening for T1D
Screening for T1D is not recommended, because individuals typically present with acute symptoms and elevated blood glucose concentrations. Consequently, the majority of cases of T1D are diagnosed soon after the onset of hyperglycemia.

---

[f] In the absence of unequivocal hyperglycemia, these criteria should be confirmed by repeat testing on a different day[3].

Testing for T2D in children

Incidence of T2D has increased in children, adolescents, and especially in minority groups.[11,12] The ADA recommends the following criteria for testing asymptomatic children with T2D:

1. Overweight (body mass index [BMI] >85% percentile for age and sex, weight for height >85% percentile, or weight >120% of ideal body weight) *and* any 2 of the following risk factors:
   a. Family history of T2D in either first- or second-degree relatives
   b. Race ethnicity—Native American, African American, Latino, Asian American, or Pacific Islander)
   c. Signs of insulin resistance or conditions associated with insulin resistance
   d. Maternal history of diabetes or GDM

It is recommended that evaluation of these risk factors begin at either age 10 years or at the onset of puberty, if puberty occurs at a younger age. Follow-up testing is indicated every 2 years in identified children, using fasting blood glucose as the preferred test.

Testing for prediabetes and T2D in adults

Diagnosis of T2D is often delayed until complications occur, and it is estimated that approximately one-third of all individuals with T2D may remain undiagnosed.[1] The ADA recommends that all individuals older than 45 years of age be tested for prediabetes and T2D, because age is a major risk factor for the development of diabetes.[1] Younger adults should be evaluated if they are overweight (BMI >25 kg/m^2) *and* have 1 or more of the following risk factors: physical inactivity, first-degree relative with diabetes, are members of a high-risk ethnic group, women who delivered a baby weighing more than 9 lb or were diagnosed with GDM, hypertension, low high-density lipoprotein (HDL) cholesterol (<35 mg/dL), and/or elevated triglyceride (>250 mg/dL), women with polycystic ovarian syndrome, prior evidence of IGT or IFG, other clinical conditions associated with insulin resistance (eg, severe obesity), or a history of CVD. Either fasting blood glucose testing or 2-hour OGTT testing are acceptable screening tools. If the tests are normal, repeat testing should be performed every 3 years.[1]

EVALUATION OF THE DIABETIC ATHLETE BEFORE EXERCISE

A 2004 statement by the ADA recommended that before increasing patterns of physical activity or beginning an exercise program, diabetic patients should undergo a detailed medical evaluation with appropriate diagnostic studies. The medical examination should screen for the presence of both macro- and microvascular complications and for signs and symptoms of cardiovascular, renal, and ocular disease.[13]

T2D is associated with an increased risk for CVD.[1,5,6] However, recommendations for routine screening for coronary artery disease (CAD) in asymptomatic patients with T2D,[14] aside from commencement of a moderate- to vigorous-intensity exercise program, has been questioned—based on a report on asymptomatic patients with T2D aged 50 to 75 years that showed 1 in 5 patients had silent myocardial ischemia.[15] The same study also suggested that the recommended screening algorithm of 2 or more risk factors did not accurately identify a large number of patients with test abnormalities.[15] Also, a recent report suggested that routine screening of asymptomatic diabetic patients for CAD is not warranted,[16] and the ADA recommends that clinical judgment should be used on an individual basis.[1]

The ADA has also provided guidelines for graded exercise testing (GXT). Current recommendations include a GXT before initiating a moderate- to vigorous-intensity exercise program as part of a lifestyle-intervention strategy in diabetics older than 35 years of age. Between 25 and 35 years of age, GXT is recommended if the diabetic individual either has T2D for more than 10 years, T1D more than 15 years, risk factors for CAD, microvascular disease, macrovascular disease, or autonomic neuropathy.[13]

GXT can be used for diagnostic, prognostic, and therapeutic purposes and is especially helpful for designing appropriate exercise prescription programs.[17] For example, in high-risk individuals with an intermediate probability of significant CAD, results of a GXT can provide clinical diagnostic information, particularly when used in the context of other clinical data.[17] Moreover, it is well accepted that low levels of fitness and muscular strength, as well as elevated levels of fatness, independently affect risk factors for CVD in both diabetic and nondiabetic individuals and are independent risk factors for all-cause and cardiovascular mortality.[18–21] Furthermore, in males with T2D, the presence of an equivocal or abnormal GXT is associated with a higher risk of all-cause CVD and CAD mortality even after adjusting for fasting blood glucose, smoking, BMI, hypercholesterolemia, hypertension, family history of CVD or diabetes, abnormal resting electrocardiogram (ECG), and fitness.[22] Therefore, an exercise evaluation protocol should be used to assess both potential clinical limitations to exercise and exercise capacity to allow for the development of an exercise prescription designed to improve fitness.

Exercise Testing for Adults

The treadmill and bicycle ergometer are most commonly used for exercise testing protocols. The advantage of the treadmill is that it is more representative of activities of daily living (ADLs) (eg, walking), and it incorporates greater amounts of total muscle mass, which results in higher maximal oxygen consumption (Vo_2 max) values. Although handrails are often used for balance, holding on to the handrails during exercise testing will affect the accuracy of the estimation of energetics and exercise capacity.[17] The cycle ergometer is less expensive, uses less space, and is preferable for individuals in whom balance on the treadmill may be a limiting factor.

Although numerous exercise testing protocols are available, the protocol used should be formulated according to the desired outcome measures and characteristics of the patient. The Bruce protocol is the most popular exercise evaluation procedure. It employs relatively large increases in oxygen demands per stage. Ramp protocols with more uniform increases in metabolic responses and hemodynamics are also recommended for exercise evaluation. Exercise test monitoring of heart rate (HR), blood pressure, ECG, subjective ratings of symptoms, gas exchange responses, and blood gases have all been suggested, depending on the goal of the exercise evaluation and the clinical state of the patient. The American College of Sports Medicine (ACSM) has well-defined absolute and relative guidelines for exercise test termination.[17]

Exercise Testing for Children

The principles used in either treadmill or cycle ergometer testing in adults are similar for children and adolescents. However, because children are relatively immature, they need encouragement and positive support by an experienced testing staff to obtain accurate results.[17] Although both treadmill and cycle ergometer protocols have been used in children, the treadmill is more appropriate for young children, because it requires the child to maintain the pace of the belt, rather than providing a volitional effort to maintain an appropriate revolutions per minute on the bicycle.

Other difficulties encountered during cycle ergometer exercise testing in children include the size of the bicycle, seat height, handlebar height and position, and pedal crank length. In addition, children and adults have different physiologic responses to exercise. Children have lower, absolute submaximal, and VO_2 max values (L/min) but higher, relative VO_2 max values (mL/kg/min) compared with those of adults. Although the HR response to submaximal and maximal exercise is higher in children, they have lower cardiac output, stroke volume, blood lactate concentrations, ventilation, and respiratory exchange ratios compared with those of adults.[17]

GUIDELINES FOR EXERCISE PRESCRIPTION

In order to achieve optimal benefits in health, well-being, and quality of life, exercise prescription should include programs for improving cardiorespiratory fitness, body composition, and muscular fitness.[17] It is important to encourage young people to participate in physical activities that are appropriate for their age, that are enjoyable, and that offer variety. Recently, the US Department of Health and Human Services provided the 2008 Physical Activity Guidelines for Americans.[23] The following recommendations are part of the guidelines:

Guidelines for Children

1. Children and adolescents should perform more than or equal to 60 minutes of physical activity daily.
2. Aerobic: Most of the more than or equal to 60 minutes of daily physical activity should be either moderate- or vigorous-intensity, aerobic physical activity and should include vigorous-intensity physical activity at least 3 d/wk.
3. Muscle strengthening: As part of more than or equal to 60 minutes of daily physical activity, children and adolescents should include muscle-strengthening physical activity on at least 3 d/wk.
4. Bone strengthening: As part of more than or equal to 60 minutes of daily physical activity, children and adolescents should include bone-strengthening physical activity on at least 3 d/wk.

Guidelines for Adults

1. All adults should avoid inactivity. Some physical activity is better than none, and adults who participate in any amount of physical activity gain some health benefits.
2. For substantial health benefits, adults should perform at least 150 min/wk of moderate-intensity or 75 min/wk of vigorous-intensity aerobic physical activity or an equivalent combination of moderate- and vigorous-intensity aerobic activity.
3. Aerobic activity should be performed in intervals of at least 10 minutes, and preferably, it should be divided throughout the week.
4. For additional and more extensive health benefits, adults should increase their aerobic physical activity to 300 min/wk of moderate-intensity or 150 min/wk of vigorous-intensity aerobic physical activity or an equivalent combination of moderate- and vigorous-intensity activity. Additional health benefits are gained by engaging in physical activity beyond this amount.
5. Adults should also perform muscle-strengthening activities that are moderate or high intensity and involve all major muscle groups on 2 or more days a week, because these activities provide additional health benefits.

Guidelines for Older Adults

The guidelines for adults also apply to older adults. In addition, the following guidelines are specifically for older adults:

1. When older adults cannot perform 150 minutes of moderate-intensity aerobic activity a week because of chronic conditions, they should try and be physically active to the best of their ability.
2. Older adults should perform exercises that maintain or improve balance if they are at increased risk for falls.
3. Older adults should determine their level of effort for physical activity relative to their level of fitness.
4. Older adults with chronic conditions should understand their limitations in performing regular physical activity safely.

Guidelines for Safe Physical Activity

To perform physical activity safely and reduce the risk of injuries and other adverse events, individuals should be educated on and adhere to the following principles:

1. Understand the risks and yet be confident that physical activity is safe for almost everyone.
2. Choose to perform types of physical activity that are appropriate for their current fitness level and health goals, because some activities are safer than others.
3. Increase physical activity gradually over time as needed to meet guidelines or health goals.
4. Inactive people should "start low and go slow" by gradually increasing frequency and time of exercise.
5. Protect themselves by using appropriate gear and sports equipment, exercise in safe environments, follow rules and policies, and make sensible choices about when, where, and how to be active.
6. People with chronic conditions and symptoms should consult their health care provider regarding appropriate types and amounts of activity.

Guidelines for Adults with Disabilities

1. Adults with disabilities, who are able to, should perform at least 150 min/wk of moderate-intensity or 75 min/wk of vigorous-intensity aerobic activity or an equivalent combination of moderate- and vigorous-intensity aerobic activity. Aerobic activity should be performed in episodes of at least 10 minutes, and preferably, it should be divided throughout the week.
2. Adults with disabilities, who are able to, should also perform muscle-strengthening activities of moderate or high intensity that involve all major muscle groups on 2 or more days per week, as these activities provide additional health benefits.
3. When adults with disabilities are not able to meet the guidelines, they should engage in regular physical activity according to their abilities and should avoid inactivity.
4. Adults with disabilities should consult their health care provider regarding appropriate types and amounts of activity.

Guidelines for People with Chronic Medical Conditions

1. Adults with chronic conditions obtain important health benefits from regular physical activity.
2. When adults with chronic conditions perform physical activity within the limits of their abilities, physical activity is safe.
3. Adults with chronic conditions should consult their health care provider regarding appropriate types and amounts of activity.

PRINCIPLES OF EXERCISE PRESCRIPTION

There exists an art and a science to thorough, meaningful exercise prescription. We recommend that an exercise physiologist be involved in developing appropriate programs for both prediabetic and diabetic individuals. All prescribed exercise programs (*conditioning* phase), should be preceded by a *warm-up* phase and followed by a *cool-down* phase. Exercises during these phases should involve large muscle, low-intensity activity and stretching. Other recommended activities may include either yoga or relaxation training. The conditioning phase should be designed to improve both cardiorespiratory fitness (VO_2 max) and local muscle fitness (blood lactate response to exercise).[17,24] Components of a thorough prescription for the conditioning phase should detail advice for exercise duration, intensity, frequency, mode, rate of progression, and specificity. Finally, training programs that use both upper-extremity and lower-extremity exercises should be prescribed.

Cardiorespiratory Exercise Prescription

Exercise duration
For most cardiorespiratory programs, the ACSM recommends 20 to 60 minutes of either continuous or intermittent exercise. For individuals who have difficulty exercising continuously, recent data have indicated that multiple bouts of shorter-duration exercise can provide similar benefits as one continuous bout of exercise.[25–27]

Exercise intensity
Exercise of an appropriate intensity is key for improvement in cardiorespiratory fitness. The combination of exercise intensity and duration determines caloric expenditure during exercise. The determination of exercise intensity is dependent upon the health and fitness status of the individual. ACSM recommends exercise intensity of 40/50 to 85% of oxygen uptake reserve (VO_2 reserve is the difference between VO_2 max and resting oxygen consumption).[17] Because oxygen consumption is not always measured during exercise evaluation programs, percentages of heart rate reserve and percentages of estimated maximal heart rate (HR) are often used as surrogate makers of VO_2 max. ACSM recommends 40/50 to 85% of HR reserve (HR reserve is calculated as the difference between HR max and resting HR times the desired training intensity + resting heart rate) or 64/70% to 94% of maximal HR (maximal HR can be estimated by subtracting the patients age from 220) for exercise prescription. For low-fit or de-conditioned individuals the lower portion of the ranges are recommended initially (eg, 40–50% of VO_2 max or HR reserve, 64–70% of age predicted maximal HR) and intensity can be increased as fitness improves. For most individuals exercise intensities of corresponding to 60–80% of HR reserve or 77–90% of age predicted maximal HR will result in improved cardiorespiratory fitness provided that frequency and duration of exercise are adequate.[17] It should be noted that the estimation of maximal HR is quite variable with one standard deviation associated with the equation 220-age being ~10 to 12 beats per minute. In addition, use of medications such as b-blockers, preclude the use of HR for exercise prescription.

Ratings of perceived exertion (RPE) are also useful for exercise prescription. The most common RPE scale was developed by Gunnar Borg[28] and is shown below:

6
7 Very, very light
8
9 Very light
10

11 Fairly light
12
13 Somewhat hard
14
15 Hard
16
17 Very hard
18
19 Very, very hard
20

ACSM recommends RPE values of 12 to 16 for exercise prescription designed to improve cardiorespiratory fitness.[17] Another advantage of using the RPE scale is that RPE are reasonable markers of the blood lactate response to exercise with the lactate threshold being associated with RPE values of ~10 to 12 and blood lactate concentrations of 4.0 mM being associated with RPE of ~15 to 17.[29,30] Similar to the use of HR there is considerable variability in RPE among individuals.

Exercise frequency

ACSM recommends an exercise frequency of 3 to 5 days per week.[17] For those exercising at the higher end of the exercise intensity range 3 days per week (every other day) is sufficient to improve (or maintain) VO_2 max. For those at the lower end of the exercise intensity range, exercise more than 3 times per week (eg, 5 × weekly) may be needed. For those individuals who are interested in exercising 5 to 6 days per week and can exercise at the higher end of the exercise intensity continuum a hard easy hard easy regimen of intensity should be applied (eg, M, W, F, high intensity; T, Th, S, low intensity) to avoid overtraining and overuse injuries.

Exercise mode

The most effective modes of exercise to improve cardiorespiratory fitness involve the recruitment of large muscle groups in rhythmic aerobic forms of activity. Activities such as walking, hiking, jogging, running, cycling, swimming, elliptical machines, rowing, dancing, skating, cross-country skiing, and aerobic games such as ultimate Frisbee have all been used to improve cardiorespiratory fitness. Sports such as racquetball, handball, soccer, and basketball are also effective provided they are played at high intensity for an adequate duration.[17] Individual likes and dislikes as well as capabilities should be taken into consideration to avoid boredom-related noncompliance with exercise programs.

Exercise progression

Exercise progression is dependent on the functional capacity, medical status, and goals of each individual. At the onset of an exercise program, there will be an initial conditioning stage in which improvements will be observed because of the transition from sedentary behavior to regular exercise. This phase is critical to preparing the individual, both for the musculoskeletal stress of exercise and to develop a lifetime approach to exercise. Therefore, during the first 6 weeks, the conditioning phase should be preceded by a longer warm-up phase and should incorporate activities designed to minimize muscle soreness, discomfort, and injury. Exercise intensity should be gradually increased during the first 6 weeks to minimize dropout.

Between 6 weeks and 6 months, or even up to 1 year, exercise frequency and duration are increased, followed by a gradual increase in exercise intensity. Finally, individuals should be transitioned to the maintenance phase after they have met their fitness goals associated with consistent levels of exercise duration, intensity, and frequency needed to maintain cardiorespiratory fitness.[17]

Specificity of training

Although most rhythmic exercises that are aerobic in nature and recruit large muscle groups will improve cardiorespiratory fitness, muscle adaptations will only occur within the muscles being recruited. This phenomena is referred to as specificity of training. For example, if one trains running and improves VO_2 max measured on a treadmill, swimming VO_2 max will not necessarily improve.[31] Local muscle responses, measured using the blood lactate response to exercise, are affected to a greater extent by training specificity than is VO_2 max.[32] This concept should be taken into consideration when developing an exercise prescription for pre-diabetic and diabetic patients. In particular, training programs that utilize both upper extremity and lower extremity exercise should be part of the exercise prescription.

Resistance Exercise Prescription

For many years, resistance training was overlooked in favor of cardiorespiratory training for patients with or at risk for developing diabetes and CAD. However, adequate muscular strength and endurance are critical for ADLs. When muscular strength and endurance are insufficient to perform ADLs, functional independence is compromised. Therefore, resistance training is recommended as part of an overall exercise prescription and should be performed on 2 to 3 nonconsecutive days of the week.[17] ACSM recommends the following resistance training guidelines:[17]

1. Chose a mode of exercise (free weights, bands, machines) that is comfortable through a pain-free range of motion.
2. Perform 8 to 10 exercises that train the major muscles of the hips, thigh, legs, back, chest, shoulders, arms, and abdomen.
3. Perform 1 set of each exercise to volitional fatigue while maintaining proper form.
4. Although the traditional recommendations of 8 to 12 repetitions is still appropriate, choose a range of repetitions between 3 and 20 that can be performed at a moderate repetition duration ($\sim$ 3 seconds).
5. Exercise each muscle group on 2 to 3 nonconsecutive days of the week.
6. Adhere as closely as possible to the specific techniques for performing a given exercise.
7. Allow enough recovery time so that the next exercise can be performed with proper form.
8. For people with high cardiovascular risk or chronic disease (eg, hypertension, diabetes), stop the exercise as the concentric phase of the exercise becomes difficult (RPE 15–16).
9. Perform the lifting (concentric) and lowering (eccentric) phases of the exercise in a controlled manner.
10. Breathe normally during lifting because breath holding can increase blood pressure.
11. Whenever possible, train with a partner who can provide feedback, assistance, and motivation.

We recommend that the aforementioned list be modified based on recent data, which suggest that higher-intensity strength training (80% of 1 rep max [RM]) may be required for meaningful benefits in older individuals.[33]

EXERCISE PRESCRIPTION AND SPECIAL CONSIDERATIONS FOR DIABETIC INDIVIDUALS
Benefits of Regular Exercise in the Management of Diabetes

The benefits of regular exercise in the management of diabetes and other disease states associated with diabetes are numerous and beyond the scope of this review and will only be discussed briefly (for a recent review on the effects of exercise and diet on chronic disease see ref.[34]).

In several large cohort studies, high risk, prediabetic individuals who completed diet and exercise lifestyle-intervention therapy (eg, 150 min/wk of moderate intensity exercise) dramatically reduced progression to diabetes.[35–37] Importantly, lifestyle modification was generalizable across race and gender, and it was more effective than treatment with the biguanide, metformin.[36]

Exercise and increased fitness are also associated with a reduced risk of complications from diabetes complications and reduced mortality in individuals with either T1D or T2D.[38,39] Clinical benefits of regular exercise and increased fitness in diabetic patients include reduced abdominal visceral fat,[40–42] improved lipid profiles,[42] increased insulin sensitivity and decreased insulin resistance,[43,44] improved endothelial function,[45,46] reduced inflammation,[47,48] reduced blood pressure,[49] and improved hemostasis.[50] Although most exercise interventions have examined aerobic, endurance training responses, there is an emerging body of evidence that indicates that resistance training also improves outcome measures in patients with diabetes.[51,52]

Type 1 Diabetes

The ADA suggests that all levels of physical activity, including leisure activities, recreational sports, and competitive professional performance, can be performed by people with T1D who do not have complications and have optimal blood glucose control.[13] Because exercise increases insulin sensitivity, it is important that individuals with T1D adjust their insulin and nutritional needs, to exercise safely and participate in high-performance activities. It is important to regularly collect self-monitored blood glucose data in response to physical activity and, subsequently, in concert with the medical staff, develop individualized treatment algorithms to improve performance and enhance safety.[13]

Type 2 Diabetes

Exercise along with diet and medication has long been the cornerstone in the management of diabetes. A recent consensus statement from the ADA provides evidence for the effectiveness of both aerobic and resistance training in the management of T2D.[53] Current recommendations for T2D include 150 minutes of moderate-intensity exercise per week and, in the absence of comorbid contraindications, resistance training for 2 d/wk.[1]

Hyperglycemia

Exercise can worsen hyperglycemia and ketosis in T1D ketotic individuals deprived of insulin for 12 to 48 hours.[1,53,54] Prior ADA position statements for exercise in T1D individuals had called for avoidance of physical activity if fasting blood glucose levels were more than 250 mg/dL (>13.9 mmol/L) in the presence of ketosis, and that in the absence of ketosis, exercise be performed with caution if glucose levels were more than 300 mg/dL (16.7 mmol/L).[55] However, in T1D individuals with ketosis, vigorous physical activity is contraindicated. It should be noted that if individuals feel well, hyperglycemia without ketosis (urine and blood ketones negative) does not preclude exercise,[1] provided they adhere to the aforementioned guidelines of blood glucose monitoring and individualized insulin needs.

In individuals with T2D, the current recommendation to avoid physical activity with blood glucose more than 300 mg/dL, even in the absence of ketosis, is probably more cautious than necessary, especially in a postprandial state.[53] In the absence of severe insulin deficiency, light- or moderate-intensity exercise would tend to decrease blood glucose. Therefore, if an individual feels well, is adequately hydrated, and is not ketotic, exercise is recommended.[1,53]

Hypoglycemia

Acute exercise increases insulin-stimulated glucose disposal in both healthy and insulin-resistant skeletal muscles.[56,57] In individuals medicated with either insulin or insulin secretagogues, physical activity can cause hypoglycemia if modication dose or carbohydrate consumption is inadequately adjusted. The risk of exercise-induced hypoglycemia is increased if prolonged exercise is performed at peak exogenous insulin levels. It is, therefore, recommended that blood glucose levels be monitored before exercise, carbohydrates be ingested if glucose levels are less than 100 mg/dL and as needed during exercise to avoid hypoglycemia, and that carbohydrates be available both during and after physical activity.[13]

Because hypoglycemia is rare in diabetic individuals not treated with insulin or insulin secretagogues, preventive measures for exercise-induced hypoglycemia are less stringent for patients treated solely by diet, metformin, α-glucosidase inhibitors, or thiazolidinediones.[1,53] The exercise response in subjects taking pramlintide (synthetic amylin analog) or exenatide (incretin analog) has not been studied, but neither is likely to cause hypoglycemia when used as monotherapy or combined with only metformin or a thiazolidinedione.[53]

Hypertension

General exercise prescription guidelines apply to hypertensive individuals with the following special considerations:[17]

1. Exercise is contraindicated if resting systolic blood pressure (SBP) is greater than 200 mm Hg or diastolic blood pressure (DBP) is greater than 100 mm Hg.
2. Individuals with marked elevation of BP (>160/100) should not add exercise training until after the initiation of pharmacologic therapy.
3. β blockers attenuate HR response to exercise and may decrease exercise capacity, especially in individuals without myocardial ischemia.
4. Use of HR for exercise prescription is not advised for patients on β blockers. Instead of HR, an RPE scale should be used to prescribe exercise intensity.
5. β blockers and diuretics may impair thermoregulation during exercise, particularly in hot and humid environments.
6. α blockers, β blockers, calcium channel blockers, and vasodilators may provoke postexercise hypotension. Therefore, a gradual cool-down phase should be emphasized.
7. Diuretics may decrease serum potassium and increase the risk for cardiac dysrhythmias and false-positive GXT.
8. Breathe normally and avoid Valsalva maneuvers—forced exhalation against a closed glottis—during resistance exercise.

For diabetic patients who are hypertensive, recommended treatment goals are SBP lower than 130 mm Hg and DBP lower than 80 mm Hg.[1] Lifestyle therapy is recommended for patients with SBP less than 140 mm Hg or DBP less than 90 mm Hg for up to 3 months. For those who either fail a 3-month trial lifestyle-therapy intervention or have SBP greater than or equal to 140 mm Hg or DBP greater than or equal to 90 mm Hg, pharmacologic therapy is recommended in addition to lifestyle therapy. Either angiotensin converting enzyme inhibitors or angiotensin receptor blockers are recommended based on individual tolerance. If necessary, a thiazide diuretic can be added.[1]

Retinopathy

Neither aerobic training nor resistance exercise has adverse effects on either vision, progression of mild nonproliferative diabetic retinopathy, or macular edema. The risk of vitreous hemorrhage or retinal detachment is increased in individuals with proliferative or severe nonproliferative diabetic retinopathy.[53] Therefore, we recommend that vigorous aerobic and resistance exercises should be avoided in this subset of individuals.

Peripheral Neuropathy

The current recommendation for patients with severe peripheral neuropathy is to engage in non–weight-bearing exercise, such as swimming, cycling, and arm exercise. This should reduce the risk of skin breakdown, infection, and the development of Charcot joint destruction.[53]

Autonomic Neuropathy

Autonomic neuropathy is strongly associated with increased risk of CVD.[15] Therefore, it is recommended that individuals with autonomic neuropathy undergo a thorough cardiac evaluation before increasing the intensity of physical activity.[53]

Albuminuria and Nephropathy

Exercise can acutely increase urinary protein excretion. However, there is no evidence that exercise increases the rate of progression of diabetic kidney disease. Therefore, individuals with diabetic kidney disease should be encouraged to exercise.[1,53]

Dyslipidemia

In diabetic patients, exercise combined with lifestyle-therapy interventions, including medical nutritional therapy—reduction of dietary trans fats, saturated fat, and cholesterol intake—and weight loss, improves lipid profile.[1] In many diabetic patients, lipid-lowering statin therapy is added to lifestyle therapy. Generally, the aforementioned exercise prescription guidelines may be applied to diabetic patients on lipid-lowering therapy, in the absence of other comorbid conditions requiring special considerations for exercise prescription (eg, hypertension).[17] However, individuals on statin therapy may experience either myalgias, muscle weakness, or rhabdomyolysis,[58] and muscular problems occur more frequently both during and after exercise.[59] In professional athletes with familial hypercholesterolemia, 78% could not tolerate therapy with any statin secondary to myalgias and cramps.[60] Therefore, in dyslipidemic diabetic patients who engage in regular exercise, an alternative lipid-lowering therapy (eg, niacin) may be required.

SUMMARY

Regular exercise training is a pivotal intervention in the overall, multidisciplinary approach in the management of diabetes. ADA recommendations include a detailed medical evaluation with appropriate diagnostic studies before increasing physical activity or beginning an exercise program. GXT is recommended before initiating a moderate- to vigorous-intensity exercise program and in individuals older than 35 years of age. In addition, individuals between 25 and 35 years of age with either T2D for more than 10 years, T1D for more than 15 years, risk factors for CAD, microvascular disease, macrovascular disease, or autonomic neuropathy should have a GXT before exercise prescription.

Prescribed exercise programs should include both aerobic and resistance exercises and should be optimally designed to improve both cardiorespiratory fitness (VO_2 max) and local muscle fitness (blood lactate response to exercise). Key elements of a thorough prescription include exercise duration, intensity, frequency, mode, rate of progression, and specificity. Additionally, training programs that use both upper-extremity and lower-extremity exercises should be included in exercise prescriptions

Diabetics should be encouraged to formulate and balance exercise programs based on individualized insulin and nutritional needs. In T1D individuals with ketosis, vigorous physical activity is contraindicated; however, hyperglycemia without ketosis (urine and blood ketones negative) does not preclude exercise. Individuals with T2D who feel well, are adequately hydrated, and do not have either severe insulin deficiency or ketosis may perform light- or moderate-intensity exercise. The risk of exercise-induced hypoglycemia is increased by inadequate adjustment of insulin dosing or carbohydrate consumption, especially during prolonged exercise performed at peak exogenous insulin levels. Therefore, blood glucose levels should be monitored before exercise; carbohydrates should be ingested if glucose levels fall less than 100 mg/dL and as needed during exercise; and carbohydrates should be readily available both during and after physical activity. In diabetics with hypertension, exercise, as part of a lifestyle-therapy intervention program, is recommended for SBP less than 140 and DBP less than 90. Exercise is contraindicated if resting SBP is greater than 200 mm Hg or DBP is greater than 100 mm Hg, and diabetics with marked elevation or BP (>160/100) should not add exercise training until after the initiation of pharmacologic therapy. The risk for vitreous hemorrhage and retinal detachment is increased in individuals with proliferative or severe nonproliferative diabetic retinopathy, and, therefore, vigorous aerobic or resistance exercise should be avoided in this subset of individuals. Diabetic individuals with neuropathy should engage in non–weight-bearing exercise programs to reduce the risk of dermatologic and musculoskeletal complications.

Individuals with autonomic neuropathy should undergo a thorough cardiac evaluation before increasing the intensity of physical activity. Exercise does not seem to increase the rate of progression of diabetic kidney disease, and, therefore, individuals with diabetic kidney disease should be encouraged to exercise. Diabetics on statin therapy may experience myalgias, muscle weakness, cramps, or rhabdomyolysis. Therefore, dyslipidemic diabetic patients who engage in regular exercise may require alternative lipid-lowering therapy.

REFERENCES

1. American Diabetes Association. Standards of medical care in diabetes-2008. Diabetes Care 2008;31(suppl 1):S12–54.
2. American Diabetes Association. Diagnosis and classification of diabetes mellitus. Diabetes Care 2008;31(suppl 1):S55–60.
3. Expert Committee on the Diagnosis and Classification of Diabetes Mellitus. Follow-up report on the diagnosis of diabetes mellitus. Diabetes Care 2003;26: 3160–7.

4. Nathan DM, Davidson MB, DeFronzo RA, et al. Impaired fasting glucose and impaired glucose tolerance: implications for care. Diabetes Care 2007;30: 753–9.
5. Galassi A, Reynolds K, He J. Metabolic syndrome and risk of cardiovascular disease: a meta-analysis. Am J Med 2006;119:812–9.
6. Gami AS, Witt BJ, Howard DE, et al. Metabolic syndrome and risk of incident cardiovascular events and death: a systematic review and meta-analysis of longitudinal studies. J Am Coll Cardiol 2007;49:403–14.
7. Expert Panel on Detection, Evaluation, and Treatment of High Blood Cholesterol in Adults. Executive Summary of The Third Report of The National Cholesterol Education Program (NCEP) Expert Panel on Detection, Evaluation, And Treatment of High Blood Cholesterol In Adults (Adult Treatment Panel III). JAMA 2001;285: 2486–97.
8. Grundy SM, Cleeman JI, Daniels SR, et al. Diagnosis and management of the metabolic syndrome: an American Heart Association/National Heart, Lung, and Blood Institute Scientific Statement. Circulation 2005;112:2735–52.
9. Alberti KG, Zimmet P, Shaw J. The metabolic syndrome–a new worldwide definition. Lancet 2005;366:1059–62.
10. Despres JP, Lemieux I, Bergeron J, et al. Abdominal obesity and the metabolic syndrome: contribution to global cardiometabolic risk. Arteroscler Thromb Vasc Biol 2007;27:2276–83.
11. Dabelea D, Bell RA, D'Agostino RB Jr, et al. Incidence of diabetes in youth in the United States. JAMA 2007;297:2716–24.
12. Liese AD, D'Agostino RB Jr, Hamman RF, et al. The burden of diabetes mellitus among US youth: prevalence estimates from the SEARCH for Diabetes in Youth Study. Pediatrics 2006;118:1510–8.
13. American Diabetes Association. Physical activity/exercise and diabetes. Diabetes Care 2004;27(Suppl 1):S58–62.
14. American Diabetes Association. Consensus development conference in the diagnosis of coronary heart disease in people with diabetes. Diabetes Care 1998;21: 1551–9.
15. Wackers FJT, Young LH, Inzucchi SE, et al. Detection of silent myocardial ischemia in asymptomatic diabetic subjects. Diabetes Care 2004;27:1954–61.
16. Bax JJ, Young LH, Frye RL, et al. Screening for coronary heart disease in patients with diabetes. Diabetes Care 2007;30:2729–36.
17. American College of Sports Medicine. ACSM's Guidelines for Exercise Testing and Prescription. Philadelphia: Lippincott Williams & Wilkens; 2006.
18. Wing RR, Jakicic J, Neiberg R, et al. Fitness, fatness, and cardiovascular fitness in type 2 diabetics: Look AHEAD Study. Med Sci Sports Exerc 2007;12:2107–16.
19. Sui XM, LaMonte MJ, Laditka JN, et al. Cardiorespiratory fitness and adiposity as mortality predictors in older adults. JAMA 2007;298:2507–16.
20. Ruiz JR, Sui X, Lobelo F, et al. Association between muscular strength and mortality in men: prospective cohort study. BMJ 2008;337:a439.
21. Siu X, Hooker SP, Lee IM, et al. A prospective study of cardiorespiratory fitness and risk of type 2 diabetes in women. Diabetes Care 2008;31:550–5.
22. Lyerly GW, Sui XM, Church TS, et al. Maximal exercise electrocardiography and coronary heart disease mortality among men with diabetes mellitus. Circulation 2008;117:2734–42.
23. U.S. Department of Health and Human Services. Physical Activity Guidelines for Americans. Available at: www.health.gov/paguidelines. Accessed March 27, 2009.

24. Weltman A. The blood lactate response to exercise. Champaign (IL): Human Kinetics; 1995.
25. Jakicic JM, Wing RR, Butler BA, et al. Prescribing exercise in multiple short bouts versus one continuous bout: effects on adherence, cardiorespiratory fitness, and weight loss in overweight women. Int J Obes 1995;19:893–901.
26. Murphy MH, Hardman AE. Training effects of short and long bouts of brisk walking in sedentary women. Med Sci Sports Exerc 1998;30:152–7.
27. Jakicic JM, Winters C, Lang W, et al. Effects of intermittent exercise and use of home exercise equipment on adherence, weight loss, and fitness in overweight women: a randomized trial. JAMA 1999;282:1554–60.
28. Borg GA. Perceived exertion. Exerc Sport Sci Rev 1974;2:131–53.
29. Steed J, Gaesser GA, Weltman A. Ratings of perceived exertion and blood lactate concentration during submaximal running. Med Sci Sports Exerc 1994; 12:797–803.
30. Stoudemire NM, Wideman L, Pass KA, et al. The validity of regulating blood lactate concentration during running by ratings of perceived exertion. Med Sci Sports Exerc 1996;28:490–5.
31. McArdle WD, Magel JR, Delio DJ. Specificity of run training on VO2max and heart rate changes during running and swimming. Med Sci Sports Exerc 1978;10:16–20.
32. Pierce EF, Weltman A, Seip RL, et al. Effects of specificity of training on the lactate threshold and VO_2 peak. Int J Sports Med 1990;11:267–72.
33. Sullivan DH, Roberson PK, Johnson LE, et al. Effects of muscle strength training and testosterone in frail elderly males. Med Sci Sports Exerc 2005;1664–72.
34. Roberts CK, Barnard RJ. Effects of exercise and diet on chronic disease. J Appl Phys 2005;98:3–30.
35. Pan XR, Li GW, Hu YH. Effects of diet and exercise in preventing NIDDM in people with impaired glucose tolerance: the Da Qing IGT and Diabetes Study. Diabetes Care 1997;20:537–44.
36. Diabetes Prevention Program Research Group. Reduction in the incidence of type 2 diabetes with lifestyle intervention or metformin. N Engl J Med 2002;346:393–403.
37. Lindström L, Peltonen M, Eriksson JG, et al. Determinants for the effectiveness of lifestyle intervention in the Finnish Diabetes Prevention Study. Diabetes Care 2008;31:857–62.
38. Moy CS, Songer TJ, LaPorte RE, et al. Insulin-dependent diabetes mellitus, physical activity and death. Am J Epidemiol 1993;137:74–81.
39. Church TS, LaMonte MJ, Barlow CE, et al. Cardiorespiratory fitness and body mass index as predictors of cardiovascular disease mortality among men with diabetes. Arch Intern Med 2005;18:2114–20.
40. Lee S, Kuk JL, Davidson LE, et al. Exercise without weight loss is an effective strategy for obesity reduction in obese individuals with and without Type 2 diabetes. J Appl Phys 2005;99:1220–5.
41. Lehmann R, Vokac A, Niedermann K, et al. Loss of abdominal fat and improvement of the cardiovascular risk profile by regular moderate exercise training in patients with NIDDM. Diabetologia 1995;38:1313–9.
42. Giannopoulou I, Ploutz-Snyder LL, Carhart R, et al. Exercise is required for visceral fat loss in postmenopausal women with type 2 diabetes. J Clin Endocrinol Metab 2005;90:1511–8.
43. Mayer-Davis EJ, D'Agostino R, Karter AJ, et al. Intensity and amount of physical activity in relation to insulin sensitivity - The Insulin Resistance Atherosclerosis Study. JAMA 1998;279:669–74.

44. Suminski RR, Utter AC. Effect of exercise intensity on glucose and insulin metabolism in obese individuals and obese NIDDM patients. Diabetes Care 1996;19: 341–9.
45. De Filippis E, Cusi K, Ocampo G, et al. Exercise-induced improvement in vasodilatory function accompanies increased insulin sensitivity in obesity and type 2 diabetes mellitus. J Clin Endocrinol Metab 2006;12:4903–10.
46. Fuchsjager-Mayrl G, Pleiner J, Wiesinger GF, et al. Exercise training improves vascular endothelial function in patients with type 1 diabetes. Diabetes Care 2002;10:1795–801.
47. Jae SY, Heffernan KS, Lee MK, et al. Relation of cardiorespiratory fitness to inflammatory markers, fibrinolytic factors, and lipoprotein(a) in patients with type 2 diabetes mellitus. Am J Cardiol 2008;102:700–3.
48. Petersen AMW, Pedersen BK. The anti-inflammatory effects of exercise. J Appl Phys 2005;98:1154–62.
49. Stewart KJ. Role of exercise training on cardiovascular disease in persons who have type 2 diabetes and hypertension. Cardiol Clin 2004;22:569–86.
50. Hamdy O, Ledbury S, Mullooly C, et al. Lifestyle modification improves endothelial function in obese subjects with the insulin resistance syndrome. Diabetes Care 2003;26:2119–25.
51. Dunstan DW, Daly RM, Owen N, et al. High-intensity resistance training improves glycemic control in older patients with type 2 diabetes. Diabetes Care 2002;25: 1729–36.
52. Ibanez J, Izquierdo M, Arguelles N, et al. Twice-weekly progressive resistance training decreases abdominal fat and improves insulin sensitivity in older men with type 2 diabetes. Diabetes Care 2005;28:662–7.
53. Sigal RJ, Kenny GP, Wasserman DH, et al. Physical activity/exercise and type 2 diabetes: a consensus statement from the American Diabetes Association. Diabetes Care 2006;29:1433–8.
54. Berger M, Berchtold P, Cuppers HJ, et al. Metabolic and hormonal effects of muscular exercise in juvenile diabetes. Diabetologia 1977;13:355–65.
55. Zinman B, Ruderman N, Campaigne BN, et al. Physical activity/exercise and diabetes mellitus. Diabetes Care 2003;26(Suppl 1):S73–7.
56. DeFronzo RA, Ferrannini E, Sato Y, et al. Synergistic interaction between exercise and insulin on peripheral glucose uptake. J Clin Invest 1981;68:1468–74.
57. Richter EA, Garetto LP, Goodman MN, et al. Muscle glucose metabolism following exercise in the rat: increased sensitivity to insulin. J Clin Invest 1982; 69:785–93.
58. Ucar M, Mjorndal T, Dahlqvist R. HMG-CoA reductase inhibitors and myotoxicity. Drug Saf 2000;22:441–57.
59. Franc S, Dejager S, Bruckert E, et al. A comprehensive description of muscle symptoms associated with lipid-lowering drugs. Cardiovasc Drugs Ther 2003; 17:459–65.
60. Sizinger H, O'Grady J. Professional athletes suffering from familial hypercholesterolemia rarely tolerate statin treatment because of muscular problems. Br J Clin Pharmacol 2004;57:525–8.

Common Injuries in Athletes with Obesity and Diabetes

Robert P. Wilder, MD, FACSM*, Michael Cicchetti, MD

KEYWORDS

- Obesity • Diabetes • Musculoskeletal injuries
- Disability • Exercise

Musculoskeletal injuries and diseases are common in persons with obesity and diabetes mellitus. High body mass index (BMI)[1] is associated with an increased risk for musculoskeletal injuries, diseases, and disability.[2,3] There is a significant positive correlation between the level of obesity and musculoskeletal injuries,[4] and disability and health-related costs. The prevalence of obesity and diabetes is inversely proportional to health-related quality of life (QOL).

Most research has focused on the effects of obesity on bone and joint problems; however, emerging data show that obesity has deleterious effects on soft connective tissue structures such as cartilage, fascia, and tendons.[5] Obesity has been associated with overuse syndromes (eg, plantar fasciitis, carpal tunnel syndrome), work-related injury and disability (eg, low back pain), injuries in children, osteoarthritis (OA), osteoporosis and fractures, gait difficulty, diffuse idiopathic skeletal hyperostosis, gout, fibromyalgia, and rheumatoid arthritis.[2] Similarly, individuals with diabetes are more prone to tendinopathies, hand and foot injuries, osteoporosis, fractures, and cartilage injury.

Exercise is an important and effective intervention for individuals with diabetes. Individuals with type 1 diabetes (T1D) who exercise regularly have a lower incidence of macrovascular disease, neuropathy, and nephropathy.[6] In individuals with type 2 diabetes (T2D), exercise has been shown to lower glucose levels, improve insulin action, and reduce overall risk for coronary heart disease. Yet, complications in T1D and T2D increase risk for musculoskeletal injuries. For example, secondary to changes in microvascular flow,[7] individuals with T1D are more susceptible to chronic exertional compartment syndrome.[8] In individuals with T2D, complications including diabetic nephropathy and retinopathy are associated with decreased capacity for exercise, as measured by maximal oxygen consumption (VO_2 max).[9] Decreased exercise performance can thus reduce a patient's ability to perform the activities of daily living and potentially enhance the risk of overuse injuries.

Department of Physical Medicine and Rehabilitation, University of Virginia, 545 Ray C. Hunt Drive, Suite 310, Charlottesville, VA 22908, USA
* Corresponding author.
E-mail address: rpw4n@virginia.edu (R.P. Wilder).

Clin Sports Med 28 (2009) 441–453
doi:10.1016/j.csm.2009.02.007
0278-5919/09/$ – see front matter © 2009 Elsevier Inc. All rights reserved.

sportsmed.theclinics.com

In the daily practice of sports medicine, medical professionals frequently encounter obese and diabetic patients with various musculoskeletal injuries and diseases. This issue reviews common injuries and diseases in individuals with obesity and diabetes. Detailed discussions on all injuries and diseases, and treatment algorithms for various injuries and diseases, are beyond the scope of this article. Evidence-based data is presented on the demographics and pathophysiologic mechanisms of common injuries and diseases observed in individuals with obesity and diabetes. This information may be used by medical professionals to devise appropriate and individualized preventive and clinical musculoskeletal rehabilitation therapeutic programs.

OBESITY: MUSCULOSKELETAL INJURY AND DISEASE
Demographics, Morbidity, and Cost of Obesity

There is a growing awareness of the long-term health complications associated with obesity. The World Health Organization has estimated that ~1 billion individuals worldwide are overweight and that 30% of these individuals meet the criteria for obesity.[2] One in 7 children and adolescents in the United States are obese and have decreased health-related QOL compared with healthy peers and a health-related QOL similar to those with cancer. Furthermore, there is a significant inverse correlation between obesity and physical functioning.[10]

Matter and colleagues reviewed discharge records of 160,707 obese patients from the 2002 Nationwide Inpatient Sample of the Healthcare Cost and Utilization Project. Demographic and injury characteristics between obese and nonobese hospitalized patients revealed that the type and cause of injury requiring hospitalization were significantly associated with obesity ($P < .001$). Musculoskeletal conditions that required hospitalization – including sprains, strains, dislocations, injuries secondary to overexertion, falls, and poisonings – were more common among obese (compared with nonobese) patients.[11]

A 3-year review of 40,304 adults from a database of the Medical Expenditure Panel Survey (1999–2002) demonstrated a significant correlation between BMI and probability of injury, including strains, sprains, dislocations, and lower extremity fractures. The odds of sustaining an injury ranged from 15% in overweight individuals to 48% in those with Class III obesity.[1]

Elevated BMI is associated with increased workplace injury, and obese workers typically report a greater incidence of work-restricting pain in the neck, back, and lower extremities.[12] Traumatic injuries were recorded over a 2-year period in 7,690 workers at an aluminum manufacturing company in the United States. Twenty-nine percent of all workers sustained at least 1 injury, and 85% of those injured were either overweight or obese. Compared with the group with ideal BMI, the odds of injury in the highest obesity group was 2.21, even after adjustment for several variables including age, gender, level of education, smoking, and job characteristics (eg, job physical demands, factory location, and time spent on the job). Injuries to the lower extremities (leg and knee) were more common in the highest obesity group.[13]

Obese individuals also seem more likely to file worker compensation claims for job-related injuries. In a cohort of 11,728 health care and university employees, individuals with Class III obesity (BMI ≥40) had 11.65 claims per 100 full-time equivalents (FTEs) compared with 5.80 per 100 FTEs for those employees with ideal BMI. Other significant effects in the same cohort of obese individuals compared with those of recommended body weight, included lost workdays (183.63 versus 14.19 per 100 FTEs), costs of medical claims ($51,091 versus $7,503 per 100 FTEs), and costs associated with indemnity claims ($59,178 versus $5,396 per 100 FTEs). Claims were higher for injuries of the lower extremities, wrist or hand, low back, inflammation, strains, sprains, contusions, bruises, lifting, slips, and falls.[14]

The Impact of Childhood Obesity and the Development of Musculoskeletal Injuries

Musculoskeletal disorders are more common in obese adults than in obese children, and the data regarding the influence of obesity and altered biomechanical function on motor performance (eg, movement, muscular strength, and balance) is sparce.[15] Despite this paucity of data, childhood obesity has been linked to acute and chronic musculoskeletal injury secondary to altered limb mechanics associated with functional and structural limitations.

Structural differences identified in obese children compared with those of normal weight include reduced femoral anteversion, increased Q angle and flatter feet.[5,15] In a study that examined the effects of obesity on foot pressure in prepubescent children, rear-foot pressure experienced by obese and nonobese individuals did not differ. However, mean peak dynamic forefoot pressure generated by obese subjects was significantly higher ($P < .001$) compared with nonobese subjects, which may negatively impact on participation in physical activity by obese children.[16]

Obese Children have also been noted to have increased medial knee compartment compression, rear foot motion, forefoot abduction, altered proprioception, and decreased balance and dynamic stability during gait.[5,15,17,18] Balance scores are negatively correlated with BMI, body weight, percentage fat, and total fat mass in obese children and adolescents'.[19] Dynamic stability is decreased compared with nonobese peers, which has been postulated to be caused by excess weight without underlying postural instability.[20] It is unclear, however, if the added mass of obesity leads to decreased stability or if the greater adiposity of the obese is the consequence of proprioceptive inadequacy (postural instability) and reduced activity.[5,15,18]

Obesity has also been linked to Blount disease (tibia vara),[21] slipped capital femoral epiphysis,[22] and children with a BMI in the $\geq$ 85th percentile for age (8–18 years) are more likely to sustain persistent symptoms (relative risk, 1.70; 95% confidence interval, 1.10–2.61) up to 6 months after an acute ankle sprain.[23]

Despite these findings, obese children and adolescents have been able to safely participate in exercise and sports. Injury during moderate physical activity and school physical education classes among high school students in the United States was not associated with being overweight, and may, therefore, provide options for overweight youth who need to increase physical activity.[24] In a cross-sectional study of 2,363 children aged between 9 and 17 years, Bazelmans and colleagues[25] showed that although obesity increased the occurrence of injuries requiring treatment, there was no association between obesity and severe injuries (those requiring hospitalization). A study of high school football players, which failed to demonstrate a significant increase in injury in obese players,[26] suggests that the incidence of musculoskeletal injuries in obese children may be reduced by regular physical activity secondary to enhanced neuromuscular and biomechanical control mechanisms.

Obesity and Overuse Syndromes

Obesity and high body mass index has been associated with tendinopathies of the upper and lower extremities. For example, maladaptive biomechanical alterations in obese individuals increases the risk of rotator cuff tendonopathy and subsequent need for surgery. In a frequency-matched case–control study of 311 patients, aged 53 to 77 years, Wendelboe and colleagues showed an association between increased BMI and shoulder surgery. Men and women with BMI $\geq$ 35 had the highest odds ratios. Trend analyses were also highly significant for men ($P = .002$) and women ($P \leq .001$).[27] In a cohort of 501 asymptomatic industrial and clerical workers, followed clinically for ~5 years, BMI greater than 30 was highly predictive for developing upper extremity tendonitis.[28]

Over a 6-year period, a study of 1,630 patients (mean age 51.8 years) with trigger digits revealed multiple trigger fingers – either 2 trigger digits in 1 hand or more than than 4 trigger digits bilaterally – only in individuals with BMI in the obese and morbidly obese categories.[29]

Obesity has also been identified as an independent risk factor for carpal tunnel syndrome (CTS). In 131 electrodiagnostically confirmed cases of CTS, BMI, in addition to anthropometric measurements (wrist ratio and shape index), was shown to be an independent risk factor for development of CTS in all patients.[30] In individuals with BMI ≥30 with electrodiagnostically confirmed CTS at baseline, reduction of BMI ($P = .0001$) over 3 months did not significantly change median nerve conduction velocities ($P > .05$).[31] These findings suggest that, aside from excess body weight, factors such as altered biomechanics of the hand and fingers potentially increase the risk for development of CTS.

In the lower extremities, obesity has been associated with several musculoskeletal injuries including plantar fasciitis, Achilles tendonitis, and tibialis posterior tendonitis and dysfunction.[32–34] Plantar fasciitis is more common in individuals with BMI greater than 30 compared with those with BMI ≤25, and reduced ankle dorsiflexion and weight bearing for prolonged periods are independent risk factors for the development of plantar fasciitis.[32] Obese individuals are also more prone to acquired flat foot (increased pronation) deformity.[35] Increased foot pronation is a risk factor for chronic plantar heel pain,[36] and in clinical practice, plantar fasciitis and tibialis posterior tendonitis and dysfunction seems to be more common in flat-footed individuals. Therefore, obese individuals with flat feet who spend most of their work day bearing their weight may be at exaggerated risk for plantar fasciitis and chronic plantar heel pain.

In a sample of 82 patients (44 women, 38 men, mean age 50 years), Achilles tendinopathy was statistically more common in those with obesity. The inverse correlate between microcirculation and obesity[37] and reduced vascularity at the insertion of the Achilles tendon in individuals with Achilles tendonitis,[38] suggests a disordered vascular etiology for the development of Achilles tendinopathy in obese individuals.

Obesity and Arthritis

Obesity has been associated with OA of the upper and lower extremities. The risk of radiographic knee OA and the rate of progression of OA are increased in individuals with obesity,[39–49] and almost twice as many obese individuals report a physician diagnosis of arthritis compared with nonobese individuals.[2] The association between obesity and knee OA is positively correlated with the severity of radiographic disease and is independent of physical activity levles.[39] Obese persons of both genders are at increased risk, but there is a higher risk in obese women compared with obese men. Weight loss has been shown to have a positive impact on reduction of symptomatic knee OA in obese women.[40]

Clear pathophysiologic mechanisms that increase the risk of knee OA in obese individuals have not yet been elucidated. Factors that do not significantly affect the association between OA and obesity include, serum uric acid, chondrocalcinosis, age, serum lipids or body fat distribution, blood glucose or diabetes, blood pressure, smoking, estrogen replacement therapy, or hysterectomy.[50] Although knee OA is associated with varus malalignment,[50] the link between obesity and hand OA suggests that other factors beyond weight bearing and increased joint stress, such as hormonal influences secondary to excessive adipose tissue, may alter cartilage metabolism.[47] Obese women have significant tibial bone enlargement and cartilage defects, without volume or thickness loss, compared with their nonobese counterparts.[51] Increased BMI correlates strongly with increased biomarkers of cartilage turnover, as well as oligomeric matrix protein and urinary degradation products of type 2 collagen.[52,53]

Other notable, miscellaneous disorders linked to obesity include bilateral, not unilateral, hip OA,[54] an increased risk for pulmonary embolism following total hip and total knee arthroplasty,[55] diffuse idiopathic skeletal hyperostosis, (perhaps secondary to increased leptin levels,[2,56]) rheumatoid arthritis,[57] gait disturbance (secondary to inadequate trunk sway and postural instability,[58,59]) and gouty arthritis.[60] Because the amount of visceral fat is a strong determinant of uric acid levels and clearance, weight reduction should be an important part of the treatment of patients with obesity and gout.

Low Back Pain

The link between obesity and lower back pain is unclear. Whereas some reports have indicated a moderate association between increased BMI and low back pain,[61,62] others have not shown a well-defined link.[63] Although overweight individuals have decreased signal intensity of the nucleus pulposus on MRI[64] and increased radicular signs and symptoms,[65] it is unclear whether these MRI findings correlate with clinical symptoms. In addition, spinal epidural lipomatosis (hypertrophy of the epidural adipose tissue) associated with obesity,[66] may mimic disc disease and produce radicular symptoms by narrowing the spinal and neuroforaminal canals and compression of related neural structures.

Conservative treatment is typically favorable in ~75% of patients with sciatica, yet obesity, in addition to heavy labor, is associated with adverse outcomes at 6 months.[67] Weight reduction following vertical banded gastroplasty reduces functional disability,[68] the use of pain medication, and persistence of low back pain. Therefore, weight reduction should be a cornerstone in the management of obese individuals with low back pain.

Fractures and Trauma

Increased BMI is associated with a reduced risk of hip and wrist fractures in elderly individuals. The mechanism of the reduced fracture rate in obese adults is not fully understood, but may be attributed to greater regional bone densities in the obese as well as a cushioning effect of adiposity during falls.[5,15] In contrast, obesity has been associated with a greater risk of distal forearm and wrist fractures in children.[5,15,69,70] Overweight and obese children have lower bone mass and area for their weight than children of normal adiposity,[55] and it has been proposed that low bone mineral content in overweight children is reflective of lifestyle factors that do not promote optimum bone evolution.[5,15,71]

Despite the protective effects of obesity on bone mineral density,[72] obese victims of blunt trauma are more likely to have rib, pelvic, and extremity fractures, pulmonary contusions, and less likely to have head trauma and liver injuries compared with nonobese victims.[73] Obesity is also reported to be a risk factor for elbow and ankle fractures requiring surgical treatment.[74] Severely overweight individuals with BMI greater than 31 have a higher rate of complications following trauma – especially pulmonary – and have a higher mortality rate.[75] Knee dislocation in obese patients is more common following low velocity trauma, including simple falls and noncontact sports.[76]

DIABETES: MUSCULOSKELETAL INJURY AND DISEASE
Special Considerations

The overall risk for persons with diabetes for musculoskeletal injury has not been extensively studied. However, compared with healthy individuals, persons with T1D have an increased incidence of certain types of musculoskeletal injuries and diseases. Diabetics tend to have delayed healing patterns, and as a result, have higher morbidity following injury and treatment.

In the absence of coronary heart disease, complications from T2D, including diabetic retinopathy, neuropathy, microalbuminuria, and overt albuminuria are associated with a lower peak VO_2. Significant independent associations have also been demonstrated between diabetic nephropathy, retinopathy, and exercise capacity after controlling for BMI, length of diagnosed disease, age, gender, hypertension, and race. Diabetics with underlying coronary heart disease and autonomic neuropathy are more prone to arrhythmias and adverse cardiac events.[77] Thus, microvascular disease reduces exercise capacity,[9] which has important implications in the development, rehabilitation, and healing of musculoskeletal injury and disease.

There is also evidence that diabetic complications, including neuropathy and vascular disease, may affect patterns of musculoskeletal injury and disease. Specifically, relationships have been identified between T1D and tendinopathy, hand and foot disorders, osteoporosis and fractures, cartilage injury, and an increased rate of complications following trauma and surgery.[77] In addition, occlusive vascular disease can cause idiopathic muscle infarction of the thigh in persons with poorly controlled diabetes.[7] Therefore, when treating diabetic individuals, clinicians should be vigilant to the uniqueness of musculoskeletal injury and disease patterns, and work with their patients proactively to identify potential problems.[6,9,77,78] For example, proper foot care is a pivotal intervention. Shoes should fit comfortably and regular skin inspection with expeditious treatment of skin lesions is a cornerstone in management to prevent development of infection. Diabetics with severe neuropathy should be prescribed non–weight-bearing exercises.[77] A thorough hands-on approach is imperative to reduce morbidity and promote healthy living in this patient population.

Tendinopathy

There is a higher incidence of tendinopathies of the Achilles, shoulder, and hand flexor tendons in diabetics.[79–82] Achilles tendinopathy is statistically more common in individuals with diabetes mellitus who are younger than 44 years of age.[34] Ultrasound evaluation of Achilles tendons in diabetics has demonstrated disorganized tendon fibers and calcifications that were more pronounced in older diabetics.[82] Electron microscopy has identified highly disorganized and increased packing density of collagen fibrils, decreased fibrillar diameter, and abnormal fibril morphology. These structural changes may reflect a poorly defined process of structural reorganization secondary to nonenzymatic glycation expressed over many years.[81] Eventually, this may contribute to stiffening and shortening of the Achilles tendon, resulting in foot problems such as diabetic pressure ulcers of the foot, stress fractures, or Charcot joints.[81,82]

On shoulder anterior–posterior radiographs, an increased incidence of calcifications, consistent with calcific tendonitis, are identified in diabetics (31.8%) compared with non diabetic controls (10.3%). The highest incidence of calcifications is noted in diabetics treated with insulin for a prolonged time,[80] and the incidence of flexor tenosynovitis (FTS) is high in diabetics, which correlates positively with the duration of diabetes. The incidence of FTS did not correlate with metabolic control or complications of diabetes.[83] Therefore, aside from the connective tissue alterations mentioned earlier, the exact cause of increased incidence of tendonitis in diabetics is undefined thus far.

Hand and Foot Disorders

Diabetics have a higher incidence of hand abnormalities including Dupuytren's disease, limited joint mobility, FTS, trigger finger, and carpal tunnel syndrome.[83–86] Akin to FTS, the incidence of these injuries increases with the duration of diabetes, and poor metabolic control does not correlate with incidence. Yet, the incidence of hand injuries increases with advancing age in those involved in heavy manual labor, and complication rates are higher following surgical correction.[83] Furthermore, the pathology is more marked in insulin-dependent diabetics.[87]

Several foot musculoskeletal disorders are common in diabetics, including diabetic ulcers, Charcot joints, osteolysis, septic arthritis, osteomyelitis, and fractures.[85,88] These seem closely related to the presence of peripheral neuropathy and the associated sensory blunting in the feet.[88]

Osteoporosis and Fracture Risk

In contrast to individuals with T2D who do not seem to have significant changes in bone mineral density,[89] patients with T1D demonstrate lower spine and appendicular bone mineral density compared with age-matched controls.[90–92] T1D is associated with an increased risk of fracture, although some studies have failed to demonstrate an increase in hip and Colles fractures between diabetics and controls.[77,85,89,93,94]

The risk for fractures in persons with T2D is less clear. However, T2D has been identified as a risk factor for falls and subsequent hip fractures in elderly women.[95] Proposed mechanisms for this increased risk include reduced vibration sensation and peripheral neuropathy. In addition, a decreased risk of low energy fractures has been reported in patients with glucose intolerance as measured by a 2-h oral glucose test.[96]

Cartilage Injury

Although no conclusive link has been established between diabetes and cartilage injury, morphologic differences have been noted between cadaver ankle cartilage specimens from persons with and without diabetes. The cartilage harvested from individuals with diabetes was significantly softer and more permeable than cartilage from controls, suggesting that joint pathology in patients with diabetes may be associated with compromised structural integrity of articular cartilage.[97] Ultrasound examinations of knees in patients with medial knee pain showed a higher incidence of morphologic changes of the medial meniscus in those with T2D compared with nondiabetics.[98]

Other Musculoskeletal Complications

In diabetics with poor blood glucose control, occlusive vascular disease can induce idiopathic muscle infarction of the thigh, which may be misdiagnosed as a tumor, secondary to latency of onset of symptoms.[7,99] Pathologic tissue alterations on biopsy include microangiopathy, necrosis, and scarring. MRI precludes the need for biopsy and is the suggested diagnostic intervention of choice.[100] Diabetics are also more susceptible to chronic exertional compartment syndrome secondary to changes in microvascular flow and collagen metabolism.[8,101,102] In diabetics, pathologic enzymatic conversion of glucose to sorbitol[103] and enhanced capillary permeability can increase tissue swelling,[102] and prompt assessment of all 4 leg compartment pressures is pivotal for limb preservation, because neuromuscular ischemia for more than 12 hours can result in irreversible tissue damage. Surgical decompression has ~90% probability of improvement and complete recovery.[104]

Diabetes is a risk factor for infection following surgical treatment of musculoskeletal injuries. Other risk factors include age greater than 75 years, alcohol and drug abuse, remote focus of infection, severe skin disease at time of surgery, multiple trauma necessitating long-term ICU admission, and extensive soft tissue injury associated with fractures. The risk factors seen most frequently are extensive soft tissue injury associated with fractures and long-term ICU admission with multiple trauma.[105] Serious musculoskeletal injuries have also been sustained following convulsion related to insulin-induced hypoglycemia.[106] Peripheral neuropathy associated with diabetes may have a negative impact on balance and thus diminish the response to rehabilitation following ankle sprains.[107]

SUMMARY

Musculoskeletal injuries are common in persons with obesity and diabetes. Obese adults with class II obesity have a ~50% greater risk of sustaining injury and report a higher incidence of work-restricting pain, workplace injury, and disability. In the United States, 1 in 7 children and adolescents match the criteria for obesity and have decreased health-related QOL. Various structural and pathophysiologic mechanisms enhance the risk of injury in obese children. Despite the increased risk of injury, obese children should be encouraged to participate in regular physical activity, which may enhance neuromuscular and biomechanical bodily functions. Complications from prolonged diabetes affect the development patterns of musculoskeletal injury and disease, and may contribute to delayed healing during rehabilitation. Clinicians should work with their patients proactively to formulate individualized treatment plans and make their patients aware of potential complications.

REFERENCES

1. Finkelstein EA, Chen H, Prabhu M, et al. The relationship between obesity and injuries among U.S. adults. Am J Health Promot 2007;21(5):460–8.
2. Anandacoomarasamy A, Caterson I, Sambrook, et al. The impact of obesity on the musculoskeletal system [Review] [186 refs]. Int J Obes 2008;32(2):211–22.
3. Al Snih S, Ottenbacher KJ, Markides KS, et al. The effect of obesity on disability vs mortality in older Americans [see comment]. Arch Intern Med 2007;167(8): 774–80.
4. Kortt M, Baldry J. The association between musculoskeletal disorders and obesity. Aust Health Rev 2002;25(6):207–14.
5. Wearing SC, Henning EM, Byrne NM, et al. Musculoskeletal disorders associated with obesity: a biomechanical perspective [Review] [208 refs]. Obes Rev 2006;7(3):239–50.
6. Albright A, Franz M, Hornsby G, et al. American College of Sports Medicine position stand. Exercise and type 2 diabetes. Med Sci Sports Exerc 2000;32(7): 1345–60.
7. Adornato MC, Glawson S, Sadoff RS. Spontaneous compartment syndrome in a diabetic patient: a case report. J Oral Maxillofac Surg 2000;58(11):1327–9.
8. Edmundsson D, Svensson O, Toolanen G. Intermittent claudication in diabetes mellitus due to chronic exertional compartment syndrome of the leg: an observational study of 17 patients. Acta Orthop 2008;79(4):534–9.

9. Estacio RO, Regensteiner JG, Wolfel EE, et al. The association between diabetic complications and exercise capacity in NIDDM patients. Diabetes Care 1998; 21(2):291–5.
10. Schwimmer JB, Burwinkle TM, Varni JW. Health-related quality of life of severely obese children and adolescents [see comment]. JAMA 2003;289(14):1813–9.
11. Matter KC, Sinclair SA, Hostetler SG, et al. A comparison of the characteristics of injuries between obese and non-obese inpatients. Obesity (Silver Spring) 2007;15(10):2384–90.
12. Peltonen M, Lindroos AK, Torgerson JS. Musculoskeletal pain in the obese: a comparison with a general population and long-term changes after conventional and surgical obesity treatment. Pain 2003;104(3):549–57.
13. Pollack KM, Sorock GS, Slade MD, et al. Association between body mass index and acute traumatic workplace injury in hourly manufacturing employees. Am J Epidemiol 2007;166(2):204–11.
14. Ostbye T, Dement JM, Krause KM. Obesity and workers' compensation: results from the Duke Health and Safety Surveillance System [see comment]. Arch Intern Med 2007;167(8):766–73.
15. Wearing SC, Henning EM, Byrne NM, et al. The impact of childhood obesity on musculoskeletal form [Review] [138 refs]. Obes Rev 2006;7(2):209–18.
16. Dowling AM, Steele JR, Baur LA. Does obesity influence foot structure and plantar pressure patterns in prepubescent children? Int J Obes Relat Metab Disord 2001;25(6):845–52.
17. Davids JR, Huskamp M, Bagley AM. A dynamic biomechanical analysis of the etiology of adolescent tibia vara. J Pediatr Orthop 1996;16(4):461–8.
18. Wang L, et al. Proprioception of ankle and knee joints in obese boys and non-obese boys. Med Sci Monit 2008;14(3):CR129–35.
19. Goulding A, Jones I, Taylor R, et al. Dynamic and static tests of balance and postural sway in boys: effects of previous wrist bone fractures and high adiposity. Gait Posture 2003;17(2):136–41.
20. McGraw B, McClenaghan B, Williams H, et al. Gait and postural stability in obese and nonobese prepubertal boys. Arch Phys Med Rehabil 2000;81(4):484–9.
21. Dietz W, Gross W, Kirkpatrick J. Blount disease (tibia vara): another skeletal disorder associated with childhood obesity. J Pediatr 1982;101:735–7.
22. Loder RT, Aronson DD, Greenfield ML. The epidemiology of bilateral slipped capital femoral epiphysis. A study of children in Michigan. J Bone Joint Surg Am 1993;75:1141–7.
23. Timm NL, Grupp-Phelan J, Ho ML. Chronic ankle morbidity in obese children following an acute ankle injury. Arch Pediatr Adolesc Med 2005; 159(1):33–6.
24. Lowry R, Lee SM, Galuska DA, et al. Physical activity-related injury and body mass index among US high school students. J Phys Act Health 2007;4(3):325–42.
25. Bazelmans C, Coppieters Y, Godin I, et al. Is obesity associated with injuries among young people? Eur J Epidemiol 2004;19(11):1037–42.
26. Kaplan T, Digel S, Scavo V. Effect of obesity on injury risk in high school football players. Clin J Sport Med 1995;5:43–7.
27. Wendelboe AM, Hegmann KT, Gren LH, et al. Associations between body-mass index and surgery for rotator cuff tendinitis. J Bone Joint Surg Am 2004;86(4): 743–7.
28. Werner RA, Franzblau A, Gell N, et al. A longitudinal study of industrial and clerical workers: predictors of upper extremity tendonitis. J Occup Rehabil 2005; 15(1):37–46.

29. Sungpet A, Suphachatwong C, Kawinwonggowit V. Trigger digit and BMI. J Med Assoc Thai 1999;82(10):1025–7.

30. Sharifi-Mollayousefi A, Yazdchi-Marandi M, Ayramiou H, et al. Assessment of body mass index and hand anthropometric measurements as independent risk factors for carpal tunnel syndrome. Folia Morphol (Warsz) 2008;67(1):36–42.

31. Kurt S, Kisacik B, Kaplan Y, et al. Obesity and carpal tunnel syndrome: is there a causal relationship? Eur Neurol 2008;59(5):253–7.

32. Riddle DL, Pulisic M, Pidcoe P, et al. Risk factors for Plantar fasciitis: a matched case-control study [erratum appears in J Bone Joint Surg Am 2003;85(7):1338]. J Bone Joint Surg Am 2003;85(5):872–7.

33. Frey C, Zamora J. The effects of obesity on orthopaedic foot and ankle pathology. Foot Ankle Int 2007;28(9):996–9.

34. Holmes GB, Lin J. Etiologic factors associated with symptomatic achilles tendinopathy. [see comment] Foot Ankle Int 2006;27(11):952–9.

35. Van Boerum DH, Sangeorzan BJ. Biomechanics and pathophysiology of flat foot. [Review] [17 refs]. Foot Ankle Clin 2003;8(3):419–30.

36. Irving DB, Cook JL, Young MA, et al. Obesity and pronated foot type may increase the risk of chronic plantar heel pain: a matched case-control study. BMC Musculoskelet Disord 2007;8:41.

37. Wiernsperger N, Nivoit P, Bouskela E. Microcirculation in obesity: an unexplored domain [Review] [231 refs]. An Acad Bras Cienc 2007;79(4):617–38.

38. Knobloch K. Eccentric training in Achilles tendinopathy: is it harmful to tendon microcirculation? Br J Sports Med 2007;41(6):e2 [discussion: e2].

39. Felson DT, Anderson JJ, Naimark A. Obesity and knee osteoarthritis the Framingham Study. Ann Intern Med 1988;109:18–24.

40. Felson DT, Zhang Y, Anthony JM, et al. Weight loss reduces the risk for symptomatic knee osteoarthritis in women. Ann Intern Med 1992;116:535–9.

41. Felson DT, Zhang Y, Hannan MT, et al. Risk factors for incident radiographic knee osteoarthritis in the elderly. Arthritis Rheum 1997;40:728–33.

42. Felson DT, Chaisson CE. Understanding the relationship between body weight and osteoarthritis. Baillieres Clin Rheumatol 1997;11:671–81.

43. Felson DT. An update on the pathogenesis and epidemiology of osteoarthritis. Radiol Clin North Am 2004;42:1–9.

44. Lievense A, Bierma-Zeinstra S, Verhagen A, et al. Influence of work on the development of osteoarthritis of the hip: a systematic review [Review] [41 refs]. J Rheumatol 2001;28(11):2520–8.

45. Sowers M. Epidemiology of risk factors for osteoarthritis: systemic factors [Review] [63 refs]. Curr Opin Rheumatol 2001;13(5):447–51.

46. Garstang SV, Stitik TP. Osteoarthritis: epidemiology, risk factors, and pathophysiology. [Review] [92 refs]. Am J Phys Med Rehabil 2006;85(Suppl 11):S2–11, quiz S12–4.

47. Magliano M. Obesity and arthritis. Menopause Int 2008;14:149–54.

48. Zhang Y, Jordan JM. Epidemiology of osteoarthritis [Review] [95 refs]. Rheum Dis Clin North Am 2008;34(3):515–29.

49. Issa SN, Sharma L. Epidemiology of osteoarthritis: an update [Review] [60 refs]. Curr Rheumatol Rep 2006;8(1):7–15.

50. Sharma L, Lou C, Cahue S, et al. The mechanism of the effect of obesity in knee osteoarthritis: the mediating role of malalignment. Arthritis Rheum 2000;43(3):568–75.

51. Ding C, Cicuttini F, Scott F, et al. Knee structural alteration and BMI: a cross-sectional study. Obes Res 2005;13(2):350–61.

52. Jordan JM, Luta G, Stabler T, et al. Ethnic and sex differences in serum levels of cartilage oligomeric matrix protein: the Johnston County Osteoarthritis Project. Arthritis Rheum 2003;48(3):675–81.

53. Mouritzen U, Christgau S, Lehmann HJ, et al. Cartilage turnover assessed with a newly developed assay measuring collagen type II degradation products: influence of age, sex, menopause, hormone replacement therapy, and body mass index. Ann Rheum Dis 2003;62(4):332–6.

54. Felson DT, Lawrence RC, Dieppe PA, et al. Osteoarthritis: new insights. Part 1: the disease and its risk factors. Ann Intern Med 2000;133:635–9.

55. Memtsoudis S, Besculides M, Gaber L, et al. Risk factors for pulmonary embolism after hip and knee arthroplasty: a population-based study. Int Orthop 2008; [Epub ahead of print].

56. Shirakura Y, Sugiyama T, Tanaka H, et al. Hyperleptinemia in female patients with ossification of spinal ligaments. Biochem Biophys Res Commun 2000;267(3): 752–5.

57. Voigt LF, Koepsell TD, Nelson JL, et al. Smoking, obesity, alcohol consumption, and the risk of rheumatoid arthritis. Epidemiology 1994;5:525–32.

58. Messier S. Osteoarthritis of the knee and associated factors of age and obesity: effects on gait. Med Sci Sports Exerc 1994;26:1446–52.

59. Maffiuletti NA, Agosti F, Proietti M, et al. Postural instability of extremely obese individuals improves after a body weight reduction program entailing specific balance training. J Endocrinol Invest 2005;28(1):2–7.

60. Takahashi S, Yamamoto T, Tsutsumi Z, et al. Close correlation between visceral fat accumulation and uric acid metabolism in healthy men. Metabolism 1997; 46(10):1162–5.

61. Bener A, Alwash R, Gaber T, et al. Obesity and low back pain. Coll Antropol 2003;27(1):95–104.

62. Han TS, Schouten JS, Lean ME, et al. The prevalence of low back pain and associations with body fatness, fat distribution and height. Int J Obes Relat Metab Disord 1997;21(7):600–7.

63. Mirtz TA, Greene L. Is obesity a risk factor for low back pain? An example of using the evidence to answer a clinical question. Chiropr Osteopat 2005; 13:2.

64. Liuke M, Solovieva S, Lamminen A, et al. Disc degeneration of the lumbar spine in relation to overweight. Int J Obes 2005;29(8):903–8.

65. Fanuele JC, Abdu WA, Hanscom B, et al. Association between obesity and functional status in patients with spine disease. Spine 2002;27(3):306–12.

66. Fassett DR, Schmidt MH. Spinal epidural lipomatosis: a review of its causes and recommendations for treatment [Review] [19 refs]. Neurosurg Focus 2004;16(4): E11.

67. Bejia I, Younes M, Zrour S, et al. Factors predicting outcomes of mechanical sciatica: a review of 1092 cases. Joint Bone Spine 2004;71(6):567–71.

68. Melissas J, Kontakis G, Volakakis E, et al. The effect of surgical weight reduction on functional status in morbidly obese patients with low back pain. Obes Surg 2005;15(3):378–81.

69. Goulding A, Taylor RW, Jones IE, et al. Overweight and obese children have low bone mass and area for their weight. Int J Obes Relat Metab Disord 2000;24(5): 627–32.

70. Goulding A, Jones I, Taylor R, et al. Bone mineral density and body composition in boys with distal forearm fractures: a dual-energy x-ray absorptiometry study [see comment]. J Pediatr 2001;139(4):509–15.

71. Weiler H, Janzen L, Green K. Percent body fat and bone mass in healthy Canadian females 10-19 years of age. Bone 2007;37:62–5.

72. Pluijm SM, Visser M, Smit JH, et al. Determinants of bone mineral density in older men and women: body composition as mediator. J Bone Miner Res 2001;16(11):2142–51.

73. Boulanger B, Milzman D, Mitchell K. Body habitus as a predictor of injury pattern after blunt trauma. J Trauma 1992;33:228–32.

74. Bostman O. Body mass index of patients with elbow and ankle fractures requiring surgical treatment. J Trauma 1994;37:62–5.

75. Choban P, Weireter L, Maynes C. Obesity and increased mortality in blunt trauma. J Trauma 1991;32:670–1.

76. Petola E, Lindahl J, Hietaranta H. Knee dislocation in overweight patients. Am J Roentgenol 2009;192:101–6.

77. Chipkin S, Klugh S, Chasan-Taber L. Exercise and diabetes. Cardiol Clin 2001;19:489–505.

78. Graham C, Lasko-McCarthey P. Exercise options for persons with diabetic complications. Diabetes Educ 1990;16:212–20.

79. Bridgman J. Periarthritis of the shoulder and diabetes mellitus. Ann Rheum Dis 1972;31:69–71.

80. Mavrikakis M, Srimis S, Kontoyannis D, et al. Calcific shoulder periarthritis (tendinitis) in adult onset diabetes mellitus: a controlled study. Ann Rheum Dis 1989;48:211–4.

81. Grant WP, Sullivan R, Sonenshine DE, et al. Electron microscopic investigation of the effects of diabetes mellitus on the Achilles tendon. Foot Ankle Surg 1997;36(4):272–8 [discussion: 330].

82. Batista F, Nery C, Pinzur M, et al. Achilles tendinopathy in diabetes mellitus. Foot Ankle Int 2008;29(5):498–501.

83. Gamstedt A, Holm-Glad J, Ohlson C, et al. Hand abnormalities are strongly associated with the duration of diabetes mellitus. J Intern Med 1993;234:189–93.

84. Arkkila P, Kantola I, Viikari J. Limited joint mobility in type 1 diabetic patients: correlation to other diabetic complications. J Intern Med 1994;236:215–23.

85. Ramos-Remus C, Sahagun RM, Perla-Navarro AV. Endocrine disorders and musculoskeletal diseases [Review] [81 refs]. Curr Opin Rheumatol 1996;8(1):77–84.

86. Fitzgibbons PG, Weiss AP. Hand manifestations of diabetes mellitus [Review] [38 refs]. J Hand Surg [Am] 2008;33(5):771–5.

87. Chammas M, Bousquet P, Renard E, et al. Dupuytren's disease, carpal tunnel syndrome, trigger finger, and diabetes mellitus. J Hand Surg [Am] 1995;20:109–14.

88. Lisle DK, Trojian TH. Managing the athlete with type 1 diabetes [Review] [22 refs]. Curr Sports Med Rep 2006;5(2):93–8.

89. Heath H, Melton L, Chu C. Diabetes mellitus and risk of skeletal fracture. N Engl J Med 1980;303:567–70.

90. Rosen C. Endocrine disorders and osteoporosis. Curr Opin Rheumatol 1997;9:355–61.

91. Hui S, Epstein S, Johnston C. A prospective study of bone mass in patients with type 1 diabetes. J Clin Endocrinol Metab 1985;60:74–80.

92. Mathiassen B, Nielsen S, Ditzel J. Long-term bone loss in insulin-dependent diabetes mellitus. J Intern Med 1990;227:325–7.

93. Melchior T, Sorensen H, Torp-Pedersen C. Hip and distal arm fracture rates in peri- and postmenopausal insulin-treated diabetic females. J Intern Med 1994;236:203–8.

94. El-Khoury GY, Kathol MH. Neuropathic fractures in patients with diabetes mellitus. Radiology 1980;134:313–6.
95. Patel S, Hyer S, Tweed K, et al. Risk factors for fractures and falls in older women with type 2 diabetes mellitus. Calcif Tissue Int 2008;82(2):87–91.
96. Holmberg AH, Nilsson PM, Nilsson JA, et al. The association between hyperglycemia and fracture risk in middle age. A prospective, population-based study of 22,444 men and 10,902 women. J Clin Endocrinol Metab 2008;93(3):815–22.
97. Athanasiou KA, Fleishli JG, Bosma J, et al. Effects of diabetes mellitus on the biomechanical properties of human ankle cartilage. Clin Orthop Relat Res 1999;(368):182–9.
98. Unlu Z, Ozmen B, Tarhan S, et al. Ultrasonagraphic evaluation of pes anserinus tendino-bursitis in patients with type 2 diabetes mellitus. J Rheumatol 2003; 30(2):352–4.
99. Banker B, Chester C. Infarction of the thigh muscle in the diabetic patient. Neurology 1973;23:667–77.
100. Reich S, Weiner S, Chester S, et al. Clinical and radiologic features of spontaneous muscle infarction in the diabetic. Clin Nucl Med 1985;12:876–9.
101. Coley S, Situnayake R, Allen M. Compartment syndrome, stiff joints, and diabetic cheiroarthropathy. Ann Rheum Dis 1993;52:840.
102. Brownlee M. Alpha II-macroglobulin and reduced basement membrane degeneration in diabetes. Lancet 1976;1:779–80.
103. Gabbay K, Merola L, Field R. Sorbitol pathway: presence in nerve and cord with substrate accumulation in diabetes. Science 1966;151:209–10.
104. Delee J, Drez D. Orthopedic sports medicine. Philadelphia: Saunders; 1994. p. 1612.
105. Dzupa V, Dzupova O, Bendova E, et al. [Infectious complications of surgically treated musculoskeletal injuries: review of risk factors and etiological agents in years 2000–2005]. [in Czech]. Klinicka Mikrobiologie a Infekcni Lekarstvi 2007;13(6):242–7.
106. Hepburn D, Steel J, Frier B. Hypoglycemic convulsions cause serious musculoskeletal injuries in patients with IDDM. Diabetes Care 1989;12:32–4.
107. Akbari M, Karimi H, Farahini H, et al. Balance problems after unilateral lateral ankle sprains. J Rehabil R D 2006;43(7):819–24.

Hypoglycemia in Athletes with Diabetes

Susan E. Kirk, MD

KEYWORDS

• Hypoglycemia • Diabetes • Athlete • Exercise • Sport

For many years, one of the mainstays of therapy for patients with either type 1 or type 2 diabetes has been exercise, balanced with medical nutrition therapy and medications. A key limitation to achieving this balance has been the increased risk of hypoglycemia, including that induced by increased glucose use brought about by exercise or athletic activity. An absolute lack of insulin typifies the underlying pathophysiology of type 1 diabetes, whereas insulin resistance, and/or a relative lack of insulin, is more characteristic of type 2 diabetes. Until recently, children, adolescents, and young adults with diabetes who were involved in structured, competitive, athletic activity were far more likely to have type 1 diabetes. However, with the significant increase in the number of overweight or obese children and adolescents with type 2 diabetes,[1] the ratio of patients with diabetes who are involved in sports may shift. This review focuses primarily on type 1 diabetes and athletic activity; however, many of the principles discussed below apply to type 2 diabetes as well.

HYPOGLYCEMIA

Normal fasting glucose levels are defined as ranging between 72 and 100 mg/dL.[2,3] Human physiology has a number of regulatory and counter-regulatory mechanisms in place to allow both fasting and nonfasting serum glucose levels to be maintained within a relatively narrow range, despite the impact of eating, which increases serum glucose, and physical activity, which in general has the opposite effect. There are numerous other factors that significantly affect glucose levels, which may be important in exercise or athletic activity. These include stress, level of hydration, the rate of glycogenolysis and gluconeogenesis, and the secretion of counter-regulatory hormones. In addition, recent intramuscular or intra-articular injections of glucocorticoids may also significantly increase serum glucose levels.

Symptoms and signs of hypoglycemia can be broken down into 2 principal categories: *adrenergic*, caused by the release of sympathomimetic mediators, and *neuroglycopenic*, caused when an inadequate amount of glucose is available to support brain activity.[3] Both categories contain considerable overlap with symptoms caused

Division of Endocrinology, University of Virginia Health System, PO Box 800136, McKim Hall, Room 4012, Charlottesville, VA 22808, USA
E-mail address: sek4b@virginia.edu

Clin Sports Med 28 (2009) 455–468
doi:10.1016/j.csm.2009.02.003   sportsmed.theclinics.com
0278-5919/09/$ – see front matter © 2009 Elsevier Inc. All rights reserved.

by strenuous or prolonged physical activity, which may make recognition of low blood glucose difficult during athletic activity. Adrenergic signs and symptoms include hunger, anxiety, sweating, tremor, tachycardia, palpitations, and/or a feeling of impending doom. Neuroglycopenic symptoms and signs include weakness or fatigue, slow or slurred speech, impaired performance of tasks, incoordination, blurred vision, odd behavior, confusion, vertigo, paresthesias, and/or stupor.[3] Severe neuroglycopenia can lead to seizures and loss of consciousness, although these are less common in adults than they are in children.[4] Severe hypoglycemia, defined as that requiring the assistance of another person for treatment or that associated with loss of consciousness or seizures, is the most common reason for emergency room visits in patients with type 1 diabetes.[5] Any type of aerobic activity can cause signs and symptoms similar or identical to those seen with hypoglycemia. In addition, individuals engaged in athletic activity who are suffering from dehydration or heat-induced illness may have symptoms that mimic neuroglycopenia. Although people without diabetes generally do not feel symptomatic from hypoglycemia until glucose levels drop below 50 to 55 mg/dL,[3] in general patients with diabetes and intact counter-regulatory systems develop symptoms at higher levels (65–70 mg/dL). Symptoms can be felt at even greater levels if glucose values are chronically elevated above the normal range or if the rate of decrease in serum glucose is rapid.

Since glucose is the primary fuel of the brain, there are many mechanisms in place to prevent the development of hypoglycemia, both during the fasting state and during episodes of increased glucose use, such as exercise. The physiologic response to prevent or counter hypoglycemia is very complex, and a full review is beyond the scope of this issue (see[3] for a more complete review). However, in healthy adults, falling glucose levels trigger the following events. First, when glucose levels decrease to at or below 83 mg/dL, the secretion of insulin in suppressed. Since insulin normally suppresses the production of glucose in the liver and kidney, lower levels stimulate glycogenolysis in the liver and glucose synthesis, or gluconeogenesis, in the kidney. In addition, falling or low levels of insulin decrease glucose use rates in tissues other than the brain. As insulin levels continue to decrease and glucose levels fall to less than 70 mg/dL, 2 principal counter-regulatory hormones are secreted. Glucagon is released from pancreatic islet cells, and epinephrine is released from the adrenal medulla. These hormones stimulate glycogenolysis and gluconeogenesis; epinephrine also blocks glucose use in skeletal muscle, which is relevant when considering any type of athletic activity. Although glucagon and epinephrine are both secreted rapidly in response to hypoglycemia, their effects may be sustained. Finally, with prolonged and more significant hypoglycemia (serum glucose approximately at or below 60 mg/dL), 2 additional counter-regulatory hormones, cortisol and growth hormone, are released. The glucose-raising effects of these 2 hormones, although less profound than those of glucagon and epinephrine, may persist for several hours. Unfortunately, the tightly regulated release of glucagon and epinephrine in response to falling glucose levels is lost after the duration of only several years of type 1 diabetes, which adds to the difficulty of managing glucose levels during sports and exercise.[3]

Finally, there are known conditions that affect the counter-regulatory response to hypoglycemia that may be encountered in athletes with type 1 diabetes: antecedent exercise,[6] antecedent hypoglycemia,[7] and autonomic neuropathy.[8] Although it is difficult to precisely quantitate the effect of each condition when acutely managing glucose during exercise, repeated experience with these situations by the individual should help individualize any necessary adaptations to help prevent hypoglycemia.

GLUCOSE TRANSPORT AND USE IN HEALTH AND DIABETES

A key part of managing athletes with diabetes is understanding the use of glucose by skeletal tissue, both in the resting and exercising states. An explosion of knowledge of the molecular intricacies involved in this area has occurred over the past decade. However, a basic understanding of the role of the GLUT 4 glucose transport system can be helpful.[9] Glucose is transported from the blood into the cell by the GLUT family of isoformic carrier proteins.[10] GLUT4 is the major isoform that is expressed in skeletal muscle.[11] GLUT 4 expression, and, therefore, glucose transport into skeletal muscle, can be profoundly affected by a single episode of activity, and yet adaptations can also occur with chronic physical training.[9] Acute exercise causes GLUT4 to be translocated from within an intracellular compartment to the plasma membrane along non-junctional transverse tubules.[12] The resultant increase in GLUT4 transporters provides a mechanism for a constant supply of fuel into contracting skeletal tissue to compensate for increased glucose use. However, insulin also increases GLUT4 translocation in skeletal muscle; therefore, the effects of exercise can be additive or partially additive.[13] Importantly, the separate stimuli of insulin and exercise may be recruiting GLUT4 molecules from separate pools.[14] Insulin and exercise also stimulate different intracellular signaling mechanisms that influence glucose transport.[15] This increase in GLUT4 occurs both during acute contractions of skeletal muscle as well as with chronic training.[16] This physiologic adaptation explains why regular exercise can both increase insulin sensitivity and the efficiency of glucose use.

One very important aspect to consider when contemplating glucose use in type 1 diabetics who are involved in exercise or athletic activity is that often, especially in team sports, the type of activity is mixed. Exercise can be classified as low-, moderate- or high intensity, and the glucoregulatory responses to each type can be quite different. In one study, intermittent high-intensity activity (continuous exercise at 40% Vo_2 peak interspersed with additional 4-second maximal sprint efforts performed every 2 minutes to simulate team sport activity) led to greater endogenous glucose production compared with that in moderate-intensity activity.[17] The authors of the study claimed that most recommendations for managing serum glucose levels during activities do not take these different responses to varying exercise activity into account. They further suggest that insulin levels do not need to be reduced as much, if at all, during intermittent high-intensity activity.[18] Likewise, there may be a lower need for carbohydrate intake before or during this type of activity to maintain glucose levels. This recommendation is supported by the finding that subjects with type 1 diabetes who engaged in a 10-second maximum-intensity cycling sprint after cessation of moderate-intensity exercise prevented a significant fall in glucose levels.[19] In comparison, subjects who rested immediately after cessation of exercise had a further decline in glucose levels (average of 65 ± 22 mg/dL). As discussed in more detail below, each athlete should note his or her own response to these types of activity by frequent checks of capillary glucose before, during, and after activity (including, on occasion, both 90 minutes and several hours after to note a delayed response) to better anticipate his or her own unique physiologic response to exercise.

PHARMACOLOGIC THERAPIES FOR DIABETIC ATHLETES
Insulin

Patients with type 1 diabetes have little or no endogenous insulin secondary to auto-immune destruction of insulin-secreting islet cells in the pancreas. Therefore, they must use insulin to control their blood glucose levels. Although inhaled insulin was briefly available in commercial pharmacies,[20] and several pharmaceutical companies currently have oral insulin in development, at the present time, insulin is available only by subcutaneous delivery for day-to-day management of diabetes. Patients with type 2 diabetes often need higher levels of insulin to overcome underlying insulin resistance; for these patients, 1 or 2 injections per day of an intermediate- or long-acting insulin may suffice. However, patients with type 1 diabetes are likely to need a more precise regimen, with insulin delivered both continually to meet basic metabolic needs (basal insulin) and also to prevent the associated rise in glucose levels with meals or snacks (bolus insulin).

Commercially available insulin has evolved considerably over the past few decades. Until the early 1980s, insulin was purified from the pancreata of pigs and cattle, and in rare cases of insulin allergy or severe insulin resistance, salmon. With the advances of bioengineering, recombinant human insulin became commercially available in 1982 and is now the only insulin available for use in the United States. Modifications with protamine and zinc prolong the half-life of insulin so that it could be administered for basal needs.

Human insulin, when processed commercially, has a tendency to aggregate and form hexamers. Since hexamers must disassociate after injection, the onset of insulin action is delayed and its half-life prolonged, creating nonphysiologic kinetics. In the early 1990s, pharmaceutical companies began to develop analogs to the insulin. These were designed with slight modifications to the amino acid sequence of the insulin molecule, which enhanced their physiologic profiles (**Table 1**). Amino acid substitutions in the B chain of insulin prevent hexamer formation so that insulin is immediately active upon injection. Other modifications to both the A- and B- chains lead to an increase in solubility or half-life. The former has led to a more ideal delivery of bolus insulin, whereas the latter has improved the delivery of insulin used for basal needs. Recombinant human insulin also adheres to any type of plastic tubing, which is problematic for use in insulin pumps. However, none of the rapid-acting insulin analogs have this property and thus are ideal for pump therapy.

Table 1
Insulin analogs

Insulin Analog (Brand Name)	Modification of Insulin Molecule	Onset of Action	Peak Action	Duration
Modification of B chain of insulin molecule				
Lispro (Humalog)	Reversal of lysine and proline at position	5–15 min	30–90 min	1–3 h
Aspart (Novolog)	Substitution of aspartic acid for proline at position 28	5–15 min	30–90 min	1–3 h
Glulisine (Apidra)	Substitution of lysine for asparagine at position 3; substitution of glutamic acid for lysine at position B29	5–15 min	30–90 min	1–3 h
Modification of solubility of insulin molecule				
Glargine (Lantus)	2 arginine residues added to B chain; substitution of asparagine by glycine at position 21 on A chain	1–2 h	Peakless in most patients	17–24 h
Detemir (Levemir)	Lysine at position 29 on B chain bound to myristic acid	2–4 h	Peakless in most patients	~20 h; longer with higher doses

Basal-Bolus Insulin Therapy

The development of highly specialized insulin has allowed more physiologic regimens to be employed in the care of patients with type 1 diabetes. In healthy individuals, insulin is secreted continuously in low amounts but then increases sharply when food, especially carbohydrates, is consumed. One type of intensive insulin therapy, referred to as multiple daily injections, or MDI, uses a long-acting insulin, such as insulin glargine (Lantus) or insulin detemir (Levemir), injected once or twice a day, including a bedtime injection, to provide fairly constant, low levels of circulating insulin. NPH, which is a recombinant human, intermediate-duration insulin, can also be used for this purpose, but because of its property to peak at 6 to 8 hours and because of its shorter duration, it is less ideal. However, NPH is often considerably less expensive than any of the newer insulin analogs. The other component of MDI therapy includes mealtime insulin, administered as a bolus immediately before eating, preferably matched to the number of calories or carbohydrates that are to be consumed. The insulin analogs lispro (Humalog), aspart (Novolog), and glulisine (Apidra) are ideal for this purpose. These agents have a rapid absorption and onset of action and generally peak in synchrony with postprandial glucose levels. A fast-acting recombinant human insulin has been available for decades (Regular). Like NPH, it is generally much less expensive than the insulin analogs, but its physiologic properties (both a delayed onset and longer duration of action) make it less efficient for mealtime use. MDI regimens, therefore, require a minimum of 3 to 4 injections each day. When MDI regimens are used in athletes, care should be given to avoid the injection of fast-acting insulin just before exercise or athletic activity, because this may significantly increase the risk of a serious hypoglycemic event. One drawback of MDI regimens is that basal insulin delivery cannot be easily adjusted to accommodate exercise or sports. Therefore, the only option available to the athlete to prevent hypoglycemia is to consume fast-acting carbohydrates, either before and/or during the athletic activity, to prevent serum glucose levels from declining to hypoglycemic levels.

Continuous Subcutaneous Insulin Infusion—Insulin Pump Therapy

By far the most significant advance in the ability to deliver insulin intensively has been the development and increasingly widespread use of insulin pumps (continuous subcutaneous insulin infusion) in patients with diabetes, primarily those with type 1 diabetes. Insulin pumps are external devices, which can be programmed to deliver fast-acting insulin in very precise amounts, to cover both basal and bolus needs. In general, the pumps hold disposable cartridges filled with insulin, which is delivered through a small plastic catheter to a subcutaneous insertion site (**Fig. 1**). Cartridges usually hold between 1.5 and 3.0 mL of insulin (150–300 U) and must be changed every 3 to 6 days. Sites must be prepared in sterile fashion before insertion of the subcutaneous catheter, which must be changed every 3 days to avoid infection. The insertion site and pump catheter have interlocking ends that can be connected (see **Fig. 1A**) and disconnected (see **Fig. 1B**), thereby allowing the pump to be removed for short periods of time for such activities as bathing, swimming, or during intimate activities. A variety of accessories, such as sports bras or belts, have been designed to hold the pump in place during routine exercise or athletic activity, although many athletes simply wear it in a pocket or securely clipped to a uniform (**Fig. 2**). No pumps that are currently available for purchase are designed to be waterproof for long periods of time, making them a less attractive option for those who compete in water sports.

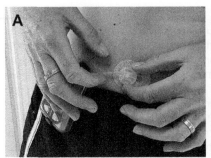 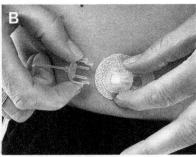

Fig.1. Insulin is delivered from the pump to the patient through a small plastic tube, which is connected to a cannula, inserted under the skin (*A*). Most insertion sets can be disconnected and reconnected at the connection hub (*B*), which is held in place on the skin by an adhesive. Subcutaneous cannulae must be replaced every 2 to 3 d. Tubing is generally replaced whenever the insulin reservoir is changed, but generally every 5 to 6 d.

Basal insulin usually comprises 50% of daily insulin requirements, which are typically 0.3 to 0.5 U/kg for normal-weight individuals with type 1 diabetes. Pumps can be programmed to deliver insulin in increments as small as 0.05 U/h. Basal rates can also be varied throughout the day, to deliver more insulin in times of decreased sensitivity (for example, during the early morning cortisol surge) or decreased insulin requirements. Most patients using a pump have 4 to 6 different basal rates in any one 24-h period. Different whole-day basal rates can be devised as well, to accommodate different insulin needs on weekdays versus weekends or to meet the insulin

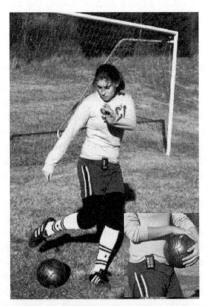

Fig. 2. Insulin pumps can be worn during exercise or athletic activity by clipping to clothing or using accessories such as specialty belts or pockets. Insulin contained in the reservoir is stable over a wide range of ambient temperatures; however, care must be taken to avoid freezing of insulin or exposing it to very high temperatures for prolonged periods of time.

needs of patients who work different shifts. The delivery of basal insulin can also be temporarily adjusted to accommodate changes in insulin sensitivity (such as those experienced during illness or at times of the menstrual cycle) or activity. Unlike injected insulin, basal insulin can either be reduced or completely suspended during exercise, which can help reduce the risk of a serious hypoglycemic event during activity. Once insulin binds to its receptor, it can remain active for approximately 30 minutes, so it may be necessary to adjust basal rates 1 half hour before beginning athletic activity. It is also crucial to remember that each athlete with type 1 diabetes has a unique response to athletic activity and other complicating factors, such as stress. Therefore, changes to insulin regimens must be developed by careful trial and error, with additional capillary glucose monitoring to prevent both hyper- and hypoglycemic responses.

Some athletes completely suspend their pumps during athletic activity, such as long-distance running, whereas others make no changes or only modestly reduce their basal rates during exercise. In a well-done study using insulin clamps to examine glucose consumption in patients with type 1 diabetes during and after aerobic exercise, 3 well-defined periods of increased glucose consumption were recognized.[21] Not unexpectedly, glucose use rates were highest both during and immediately after a 90-minute exercise period. However, glucose use rates increased again, and insulin requirements fell, 6–9 hours after the activity ceased. The authors state that most children and adolescents with type 1 diabetes are most likely to engage in prolonged athletic activity in the late afternoon, making them particularly vulnerable to a severe hypoglycemic episode during their subsequent sleep period. With this knowledge, athletes might be advised to program a temporary reduced basal night in the early morning hours after prior exercise or alternatively to increase their bedtime snack to accommodate for this phenomenon.

Although pumps can be an ideal way to tailor insulin delivery to meet the variable mealtimes and energy expenditures of athletes, health care providers who prescribe them for adolescents must consider several key issues. Several studies have shown, including one specific to children and adolescents,[22] that insulin pump therapy can allow tighter glucose control with fewer severe hypoglycemic episodes. However, despite the advantages provided by insulin pump therapy, many adolescents maintain suboptimal long-term control of glucose levels. In a study that analyzed the underlying reasons for suboptimal control in a patient population with a mean age of 15.3 years, forgetting to take mealtime boluses was the most common cause for not achieving target glucose levels.[23] Interestingly, the authors noted that 52% of the adolescents in this study disconnected their pump during exercise; however, this did not appear to adversely affect their average hemoglobin A_{1c}, a measure of glucose control over the prior 3 to 4 months (see later section). Some subjects programmed a bolus of insulin before disconnecting, but there was no comment on whether these adolescents experienced a greater frequency of hypoglycemia.

Few studies have directly addressed the use of insulin pump therapy and athletic performance. Anecdotally, pump therapy seems to be a preferred choice among serious middle- and long-distance runners, who can more easily alter their basal insulin infusion during an athletic event. There is little concern over displacement of the device or insertion site when running. However, even diabetic athletes who participate in sports with moderate contact (such as soccer or basketball) can do so successfully as long as care is given to choosing an insertion site that is less likely to come into frequent intense contact with a teammate or opposing player. Because diabetic ketoacidosis will develop after several hours without insulin, which might occur if a pump were to be discontinued for the duration of a longer sporting event, such as a swim meet or football game, the alternative use of a peakless, long-acting injected insulin, such as glargine or detemir, may be preferable in such circumstances.

Oral Agents

Although not indicated for use in patients with type 1 diabetes, there are many types of oral agents available for use in patients with type 2 diabetes. Those caring for athletes with diabetes should be familiar with their basic properties, as listed in **Table 2**. Biguanides (metformin) and the thiazolidinediones or glitazones (rosiglitazone and pioglitazone) work principally by increasing insulin sensitivity. Hypoglycemia can be seen with their use, but it is infrequent and generally mild. A third type of oral agent, alpha-glucosidase inhibitor, prevents the absorption of carbohydrates in the small intestine. The associated gastrointestinal side effects have limited its use; however, hypoglycemia is generally not encountered with this class of drug.

Incretins are newly discovered peptides, which are secreted by the gut and are known to lower glucose levels (for review, see[24]). Currently, 2 types of incretins have been recognized: glucose-dependent insulinotropic peptide and glucagon-like peptide-1 (GLP-1). Both are metabolized and inactivated by the enzyme dipeptidyl peptidase 4 (DPP4). Two GLP-1 compounds with favorable effects on appetite, glucagon secretion, and insulin production have been developed for use primarily in patients with type 2 diabetes. The GLP-1 receptor mimetic, exenatide, is available for use only by injection. However, sitagliptin, a DDP4 antagonist that prolongs the action of the endogenously secreted incretins, is available in oral form. When used

Table 2
Oral agents for use in type 2 diabetes mellitus

Class	Agent	Method of Action	Risk of Hypoglycemia	Side Effects
Biguanides	Metformin	Reduce insulin resistance in liver	Mild	Gastrointestinal; bloating, nausea, hyperdefecation, diarrhea
Thiazolidinediones	Rosiglitazone Pioglitazone	Reduce insulin resistance in fat and muscle	Mild	Weight gain, fluid retention
α-glucosidase inhibitors	Acarbose	Impairs carbohydrate absorption	None when used as monotherapy	Gastrointestinal: bloating, flatulence
DPP4 inhibitor	Sitagliptin	Prolongs action of endogenous incretins	None when used as monotherapy	Headache, runny or stuffy nose
Sulfonylureas	Chlorpropamide Glipizide Glyburide Glimepiride	Bind to receptor in islet cell; insulin secretagogue	Significant	Weight gain, allergic sensitivity in those with sulfa allergy
Meglitinides	Repaglinide Nateglinide	Increase synthesis of insulin; insulinotropic	Moderate	Back pain, headache, diarrhea

as monotherapy, it is not thought to cause hypoglycemia. Hypoglycemia has been reported when sitagliptin is combined with other oral agents.

The 2 classes of oral agents most likely to be associated with hypoglycemia, particularly during athletic activity, are the sulfonylureas and meglitinides. Sulfonylureas, which have been available for many decades, lower glucose levels by stimulating the secretion of insulin. Meglitinides are newer agents that increase the synthesis of insulin, which is then released by a natural trigger such as eating. In both cases, higher levels of insulin are present in the bloodstream, which may prevent glycogenolysis or gluconeogenesis during episodes of increased glucose use, such as exercise.

MONITORING GLUCOSE LEVELS IN DIABETIC ATHLETES
Capillary Glucose Monitoring

Significant advances have been made in the technology available for patients with diabetes to monitor blood glucose levels. Twenty-five years ago, devices to monitor capillary blood glucose levels became available for widespread use; previously, the only outpatient method for measuring glucose was in urine, which provided only a retrospective analysis of what glucose levels had been during the prior several hours. Since their first use, glucose meters have become less expensive, quicker, and more efficient. The latest generation of glucose meters works by reading the concentration of glucose from a drop of blood, which is placed on a disposable strip that has been chemically embedded with glucose oxidase, dehydrogenase, or hexokinase.[25] Meters measure both capillary blood, generally from the tip of a finger, or tissue glucose, obtained in alternative sites such as the forearm. A drop of blood is obtained by lancing the skin and placing it on the enzymatic portion of the strip. In general, a reading is available within 5 seconds, making this an ideal way to check glucose levels before, during, or after exercise or an athletic event (**Fig. 3**). Athletes should work with their health care providers or trainers to determine a safe range to maintain glucose, depending on the

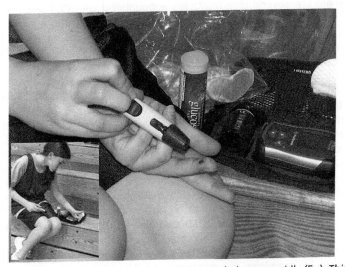

Fig. 3. Most newer-model capillary glucose monitors read glucose rapidly (5 s). This provides the athlete the option to quickly check his or her glucose level during convenient times, such as halftime or when a timeout is called. Athletes should be instructed to keep glucose-testing supplies, as well as fast-acting carbohydrates, with them at all times.

type and duration of athletic activity or exercise. In addition, they should be encouraged to check their glucose levels before the start of an exercise or activity so that any correction in low or low-normal glucose levels can be made at that time, again during the course of the activity if possible, and again at conclusion of the activity. Parents or athletic trainers should work with coaches to educate them on the need for the athlete to check his or her capillary glucose either at predetermined intervals or during breaks in play. Instructions regarding the general range in which the athlete should maintain his or her blood sugar during play (with specifications for low and high glucose levels that would cause the athlete to stop play) are also beneficial. Finally, all those involved with the athlete should be advised that he or she may need to consume short-acting glucose in the form of tablets or juice during activity either to correct or prevent mild hypoglycemia. Coaches should be taught to recognize signs of hypoglycemia, although as mentioned above, these often overlap with vigorous play.

Continuous Glucose Monitors

A relatively new development in the management of diabetes has been the use of continuous glucose monitors (CGMs). There are 2 general methods for continuous measurement. One device is designed to be worn as a watch, with a disposable pad on the reverse side that remains in contact with the skin and measures glucose continuously by a process called reverse iontopharesis. This system is no longer available in the United States. The other CGMs operate using disposable glucose oxidase electrochemical sensors that are inserted subcutaneously and remain in place for 3 to 7 days, depending on instructions from the manufacturer. The sensor communicates its readings to a monitor (or in the case of the Medtronic Paradigm, to the display of an insulin pump). Measurements are made and communicated every 1 to 5 minutes. In addition to receiving "real time" readings of interstitial glucose, most devices are also designed to record and display rate of change of glucose. These devices would have obvious advantages for monitoring glucose during exercise or athletic activity; however, there are several disadvantages encountered with their use. Importantly, none of them is completely accurate when glucose levels fall into the hypoglycemic range.[26] In addition, since the devices are measuring interstitial, rather than capillary glucose, there is an up to 20-minute lag time before the monitors accurately reflect blood glucose levels. This is especially true in the postprandial setting. Moreover, many patients with type 1 diabetes negatively view the need to wear a second external device. Finally, most insurance companies do not yet cover the cost of either the device or the disposable sensors, which are both costly.

There are limited data regarding the use of CGMs during exercise or athletic activity. One very small study (n = 6) examined the use of CGMs in subjects with diabetes who were participating in the Vienna City Marathon.[27] Although the monitors were well tolerated and did not affect the subjects' performance, importantly there was no comparison to other methods of glucose measurement. Given the meters' lack of accuracy during hypoglycemia, it is possible that some of the runners had undetected hypoglycemia. In another study examining both endurance and strength training in subjects with type 2 diabetes, the CGMs detected asymptomatic nocturnal hypoglycemia (values <40 mg/dL), which occurred with increased frequency in the post-training period.[28] In 2 cases, subjects were able to recognize patterns of diminishing glucose levels by examining the displayed results and subsequently made adjustments to avoid hypoglycemia. Clearly, there is much to be learned in the application of CGMs, which could prove to be a valuable tool in the study of exercise and its effect on glucose levels in diabetic athletes of all types.

Hemoglobin A₁c Levels in the Chronic Management of Diabetes

Hemoglobin A_{1c} is a subfraction of hemoglobin molecules that have been glycosylated over time. A higher concentration of glucose in the blood increases the chance that a glucose molecule will irreversibly bind to a hemoglobin molecule. Since the average red blood cell circulates for 120 days, hemoglobin A_{1c} levels can provide a measurement of diabetes control over the prior few months. Patients with diabetes are generally thought to have adequate control if the hemoglobin A_{1c} is between 6% and 7%. Although not practical in the day-to-day management of either type 1 or type 2 diabetes, hemoglobin A_{1c} measurements give both the patient and his or her care provider an assessment of overall diabetes control. Patients, parents, and athletic trainers should be concerned if the hemoglobin A_{1c} is very elevated (>8%), because acute episodes of exercise in poorly controlled patients with diabetes can worsen the metabolic state.

TREATMENT OF HYPOGLYCEMIA
Mild

Clearly, the best strategy regarding hypoglycemia and exercise or athletic activity is its prevention. However, it is recognized that more intensive therapy to reach target hemoglobin A_{1c} levels is associated with an increased risk of experiencing a hypoglycemic event, both mild and severe.[29] If the patient self-recognizes symptoms of hypoglycemia, or a teammate or coach suspects that glucose levels are low, the athlete should be removed from play and encouraged to measure his or her capillary glucose. Hypoglycemia should then be treated with 15 to 20 g of fast-acting carbohydrate, preferably glucose tablets designed to treat hypoglycemia or a sugar-sweetened beverage or juice. This treatment can be repeated if there is no improvement in symptoms or glucose level after 15 minutes. Foods with higher fat content, such as candy bars or chocolate, should not be used as the fat may delay absorption of the carbohydrate. Note that most beverages marketed to enhance athletic performance, such as Gatorade, may not contain an adequate concentration of sugar to quickly treat an acute hypoglycemic reaction (8 oz of Gatorade contains 14 g of carbohydrate[30] compared with apple juice and grape juice, which contain 30 and 40 g of carbohydrate respectively, in a similar volume of liquid[31]). If conditions are present that suggest that hypoglycemia might recur once the athlete resumes play, then additional complex carbohydrates should be consumed as well before returning to the activity. Those involved with assisting the athlete or person exercising should recognize that hypoglycemia provokes a counter-regulatory hormonal response, so excessive carbohydrate intake should be avoided to prevent a significant rebound into the hyperglycemic range. Finally, documentation should be made by the athlete, athletic trainer, or parent as to the conditions surrounding the hypoglycemic event, including timing of insulin injection or pump bolus, last food intake, duration or intensity of activity, or timing of the menstrual cycle, so that if a pattern is recognized, conditions can be avoided or changed for future activity. However, it is not possible to control all variables (such as mild illness or stress); despite making adjustments for all conditions, frequent monitoring of glucose levels should still be performed.

Severe

Severe hypoglycemia, involving loss of consciousness or seizures, or that which requires the assistance of another person for treatment, can be life threatening if not promptly treated. If hypoglycemia has progressed to the point where the athlete has become unresponsive, emergency response personnel should be urgently summoned. Moreover, there should be no attempt to force oral consumption of carbo-hydrates if the athlete is stuporous or has lost consciousness.

There are 2 principal methods of treating severe hypoglycemia. Glucagon can be injected parenterally, which leads to an increase in endogenous glucose production. Glucagon emergency kits can be prescribed for outpatient use, and they may be particularly useful for patients who have hypoglycemic unawareness or autonomic neuropathy, both of which increase the risk for a severe hypoglycemic event. If an athlete is prone to develop severe hypoglycemia, despite adjustments to his or her regimen designed to ameliorate the risk, it might be prudent for a coach or athletic trainer to be educated in the use of glucagon as emergency therapy.

The second method is to raise glucose by parenteral administration of high-concen-tration dextrose solution. Emergency personnel can administer 1 to 3 ampules of 50% dextrose in water (D50 W) in the field while evaluating and resuscitating the athlete. In children younger than 8 years, it is advisable to use 25% (D25 W) 2 to 4 mL/kg or even 10% dextrose (D10 W) at a dose of 0.5 to 1 g/kg.[32] Any patient or athlete requiring treatment for a severe hypoglycemic episode should subsequently contact the dia-betes care provider to discuss potential changes to his or her regimen and to devise methods to prevent a recurrence.

SUMMARY AND RECOMMENDATIONS

It is well recognized that exercise is not only beneficial to patients with diabetes but considered a cornerstone of therapy. However, exercise and athletic activity can increase the risk for hypoglycemia, including severe events, in patients with type 1 or type 2 diabetes. There are many therapeutic options available in the treatment of diabetes, including (especially in patients with type 1 diabetes) the delivery of insulin by injection or by insulin pump. Frequent monitoring of glucose, to date performed most readily by capillary glucose monitoring, can allow the athlete and his or her care provider the opportunity to analyze the effects of an exercise or an athletic activity on glucose control and to make adjustments when necessary. CGMs are relatively new devices available for patients and athletes with diabetes. With improvements in their ability to detect hypoglycemia and with changes to either insurance or the health care system to make them widely available to all patients, they may provide an ideal option for allowing real-time monitoring of glucose during exercise or a sporting event, thereby aiding significantly in the prevention of hypoglycemia.

ACKNOWLEDGMENTS

The author would like to thank Catherine Kirk Robins for her assistance with the figures and William G. Little for his editorial suggestions.

REFERENCES

1. Dabelea D, Bell RA, D'Agostino RB Jr, et al. Incidence of diabetes in youth in the United States. JAMA 2007;297(24):2716–24.
2. Expert Committee on the Diagnosis and Classification of Diabetes Mellitus. Follow-up report on the diagnosis of diabetes. Diabetes Care 2003;26(11): 3160–7.
3. Cryer PE. Glucose homeostasis and hypoglycemia. In: Kronenberg HM, Melmed S, Polonsky KS, et al, editors. Williams textbook of endocrinology. 11th edition. Philadelphia: Saunders; 2008. p. 1503–29.

4. Bognetti E, Brunelli A, Meschi F, et al. Frequency and correlates of severe hypoglycaemia in children and adolescents with diabetes mellitus. Eur J Pediatr 1997; 156(7):589–91.
5. Diabetes Control and Complications Research Group. Hypoglycemia in the diabetes control and complications trial. Diabetes 1997;46(2):271–86.
6. Galassetti P, Mann S, Tate D, et al. Effect of morning exercise on counterregulatory responses to subsequent afternoon exercise. J Appl Physiol 2001;91(1):91–9.
7. Camacho RC. Glucoregulation during and after exercise in health and insulin-dependent diabetes. Exerc Sport Sci Rev 2005;33:17–23.
8. Hilsted J, Galbo H, Christensen NJ. Impaired responses of catecholamines, growth hormone and cortisol to graded exercise in diabetic autonomic neuropathy. Diabetes 1980;29(4):257–62.
9. Goodyear LJ, Kahn BB. Exercise, glucose transport and insulin sensitivity. Annu Rev Med 1998;49:235–61.
10. Bell GI, Burant CF, Takeda J, et al. Structure and function of mammalian facilitative sugar transporters. J Biol Chem 1993;268(26):19161–4.
11. Klip A, Paquet MR. Glucose transport and glucose transporters in muscle and their metabolic regulation. Diabetes Care 1990;13(3):228–42.
12. Roy D, Marette A. Exercise induces the translocation of GLUT4 to transverse tubules from an intracellular pool in rat skeletal muscle. Biochem Biophys Res Commun 1996;223(2):147–52.
13. Wallberg-Henriksson H, Constable SH, Young DA, et al. Glucose transport into rat skeletal muscle: interaction between exercise and insulin. J Appl Physiol 1988; 65(2):909–13.
14. Douen AG, Ramlal T, Rastogi S, et al. Exercise induces recruitment of the "insulin-responsive glucose transporter". Evidence for distinct intracellular insulin-and exercise-recruitable transporter pools in skeletal muscle. J Biol Chem 1990; 265(23):13427–30.
15. Chibalin AV. Exercise-induced changes in expression and activity of proteins involved in insulin signal transduction in skeletal muscle: differential effects on insulin-receptor substrates 1 and 2. Proc Natl Acad Sci U S A 2000;97(1):38–43.
16. Karnieli E, Armoni M. Transcriptional regulation of the insulin-responsive glucose transporter GLUT4 gene: from physiology to pathology. Am J Physiol Endocrinol Metab 2008;295(1):38–45.
17. Guelfi KJ, Ratnam N, Smythe GA, et al. Effect of intermittent-high-intensity compared with continuous moderate exercise on glucose production and utilization in individuals with type 1 diabetes. Am J Physiol Endocrinol Metab 2007; 292(3):E865–70.
18. Guelfi KJ, Jones TW, Fournier PA. New insights into managing the risk of hypoglycaemia associated with intermittent high-intensity exercise in individuals with type 1 diabetes mellitus: implications for existing guidelines. Sports Med 2007;37(11): 937–46.
19. Bussau VA, Jones TW, Ferreira LD, et al. The 10-s maximal sprint: a novel approach to counter an exercise-mediated fall in glycemia in individuals with type 1 diabetes. Diabetes Care 2006;29(3):601–6.
20. WebMD. Sales of insulin exubera halted. Available at: http://diabetes.webmd.com/news/20071018/pfizer-quits-inhaled-insulin-exubera. Accessed November 28, 2008.
21. The Diabetes Research in Children Network (DirecNet) Study Group. Impact of exercise on overnight glycemic control in children with type 1 diabetes mellitus. J Pediatr 2005;147:528–34.

22. Plotnick LP, Clark LM, Brancati FL, et al. Safety and effectiveness of insulin pump therapy in children and adolescents with type 1 diabetes. Diabetes Care 2003; 26(4):1142–6.

23. Burdick J, Chase P, Slover RH, et al. Missed insulin meal boluses and elevated hemoglobin A1c levels in children receiving insulin pump therapy. Pediatrics 2004;113(3):e221–4.

24. Chia CW, Egan JM. Incretin-based therapies in type 2 diabetes mellitus. J Clin Endocrinol Metab 2008;93(10):3703–16.

25. US Food and Drug Administration. Available at: www.fda.gov/Diabetes/glucose. html. Accessed November 28, 2008.

26. Kovatchev B, Anderson S, Heinemann L, et al. Comparison of the numerical and clinical accuracy of four continuous glucose monitors. Diabetes Care 2008;31(6): 1160–4.

27. Cauza E, Hanusch-Ensere U, Strasser B, et al. Continuous glucose monitoring in diabetic long distance runners. Int J Sports Med 2005;26:774–80.

28. Cauza E, Hanusch-Ensere U, Strasser B, et al. Strength and endurance training lead to different post exercise profiles in diabetic participants using a continuous glucose monitoring system. Eur J Clin Invest 2005;35(12):745–51.

29. Ryan C, Gurtunca N, Becker D. Hypoglycemia: a complication of diabetes therapy in children. Pediatr Clin North Am 2005;52:1705–33.

30. Available at: http://www.gatorade.com. Accessed November 28, 2008.

31. Available at: http://cpmcnet.columbia.edu/dept/nbdiabetes/faq/pdf/carbohydrate_ content.pdf. Accessed November 28, 2008.

32. Cydulka RK, Pennington Jeffrey. Diabetes mellitus and disorders of glucose homeostasis. In: Marx JA, editor. Rosen's emergency medicine: concepts and clinical practice. 6th edition. Philadelphia: Mosby; 2006. p. 1955–74.

Hyperglycemic Emergencies in Athletes

Michael E. Chansky, MD[a,b,]*, Jillian G. Corbett, MD[b,c], Evan Cohen, MD[b]

KEYWORDS

- Diabetes • Exercise • Hyperglycemia • Ketoacidosis • Athletes

EPIDEMIOLOGY

Diabetes mellitus (DM) is a chronic endocrine disorder characterized by increased circulating blood levels of glucose and abnormalities in fat, protein, and carbohydrate metabolism, which can lead to longstanding macro- and microvascular complications.[1] According to the Centers for Disease Control and Prevention statistics, it is estimated that 23.6 million people, or 7.8% of the US population, are affected by DM. Among this group, roughly 185,000 are younger than 20 years of age, and 7.8 million are aged 20 to 39 years. This age group constitutes the majority of athletes and, thus, the population of interest for this discussion.[2]

TYPE 1 VERSUS TYPE 2 DIABETES MELLITUS

DM is classified into 2 major groups, type 1 and type 2. Type 1 DM (formerly known as insulin-dependent diabetes mellitus (IDDM) or juvenile-onset DM) is caused by autoimmune destruction of pancreatic islet β cells, leading to loss of insulin secretion and absolute insulin deficiency.[1] As a result, lifelong insulin replacement therapy is required for survival.[3] Type 1 DM is the most common form of the disease seen in children and adolescents, particularly of European origin.[1] As a result, the majority of athletic encounters will involve individuals with type 1 diabetes. When symptomatic, type 1 DM usually manifests with rapid onset of acute symptoms, the most severe acute complication being diabetic ketoacidosis (DKA).

Type 2 DM, the most common form of the disease (formerly referred to as non–insulin-dependent DM or adult-onset DM) is characterized by relative, rather than

[a] Emergency Medicine and Internal Medicine, UMDNJ/Robert Wood Johnson Medical School, USA
[b] Department of Emergency Medicine, Cooper University Hospital, One Cooper Plaza, Camden, NJ 08103, USA
[c] Emergency Medicine, UMDNJ/Robert Wood Johnson Medical School, USA
* Corresponding author. Chairman, Department of Emergency Medicine, One Cooper Plaza, Camden, NJ 08103.
E-mail address: chansky-michael@cooperhealth.edu (M.E. Chansky).

Clin Sports Med 28 (2009) 469–478
doi:10.1016/j.csm.2009.02.001
sportsmed.theclinics.com
0278-5919/09/$ – see front matter © 2009 Elsevier Inc. All rights reserved.

absolute, insulin deficiency.[3] Patients suffer from a combination of inadequate insulin secretion and resistance to insulin action, which may eventually lead to β cell failure and need for insulin supplementation.[4] Type 2 DM has a stronger genetic predisposition and is usually a disease of adulthood and obesity. The prevalence of type 2 DM is rising, specifically in children and teenagers.[3] Symptoms are typically less acute in onset than those of type 1 DM, and patients are less prone to ketosis but rather a hyperosmolar, hyperglycemic nonketotic syndrome.[4]

DIABETES AND EXERCISE

As previously noted, the prevalence of type 1 diabetes among children, adolescents, and young adults means this is the form of disease encountered in most athletes.[5] This discussion focuses on the management of hyperglycemic emergencies in the athlete with insulin-dependent diabetes. A review of the body's metabolic response to exercise and the physiologic effects of exercise in athletes with diabetes is important to understand the pathogenesis and therapy of DKA.

In any athlete, the primary goal during exercise is to maintain a supply of metabolic fuels for muscle and overall increasing energy needs.[6] To achieve this during states of physical activity, the body undergoes specific changes to balance glucose use by muscle and the mobilization of fuel sources from other tissues. The primary sources of fuel during exercise are divided into those present in muscle and those from extramuscular sources. Muscle sources include glycogen and triglycerides, whereas extramuscular sources include glucose released into the bloodstream via glycogenolysis and fatty acids released from adipose tissue.[7] During initial stages of exercise, muscle glycogen is used as the primary source of energy via anaerobic metabolism. As exercise duration increases, aerobic metabolism predominates, and energy is mainly derived via gluconeogenesis by the liver and release of free fatty acids.[6] This aforementioned process is regulated by a complex neural and hormonal response at exercise onset, ultimately resulting in increased plasma levels of epinephrine, decreased levels of insulin, and increased levels of glucagon, cortisol, and growth hormone (counter-regulatory hormones). Epinephrine stimulates the release of free fatty acids from lipocytes and stimulates liver glycogenolysis. A decrease in insulin secretion and increase in the counter-regulatory hormones further stimulate lipolysis and increase hepatic glucose production.[7]

In contrast to the organized process described above, the exercise response in a type 1 diabetic athlete is complicated, because normal endogenous variations in insulin and counter-regulatory hormones are absent. Instead, glucose homeostasis requires exogenous insulin administration, posing the challenge to maintain a balance between glucose level and insulin availability.[6] During exercise, diabetics may experience problems with both excessive versus insufficient amounts of insulin, leading to either a hypoglycemic or hyperglycemic state.[5] Hypoglycemia is a more frequently encountered problem and is usually a result of overinsulinization for various reasons. First, subcutaneously injected insulin is absorbed at a more rapid rate during exercise due to the increase in body temperature and skeletal muscle blood flow. In addition, the diabetic athlete does not have the ability to mount the normal hormonal response to exercise. This inability to decrease plasma insulin levels and increase secretion of counter-regulatory hormones causes a relative hyperinsulinemia, which impairs hepatic glucose production and worsens hypoglycemia.[8]

More important to this discussion is the risk of hyperglycemia in the exercising diabetic. In the normal athlete, the body responds to exercise by suppressing insulin release and stimulating release of glucagon, leading to a synergistic increase in plasma glucose levels. At rest, insulin is secreted and counter-regulatory hormone levels decrease, returning plasma glucose levels to normal.[6] In type 1 diabetics, plasma glucose levels remain elevated following periods of exercise, since there is no rise in insulin level. This absence of insulin response impairs glucose uptake and stimulates hepatic glucose production, lipolysis, and ketogenesis, ultimately resulting in a hyperglycemic state and, in the most severe cases, ketoacidosis.[9] Hyperglycemia with and without ketosis as well as the recognition, treatment, and prevention of both conditions are discussed in further detail below.

ACUTE HYPERGLYCEMIA AND KETOACIDOSIS

Acute hyperglycemia with or without ketosis is a potential hazard for any athlete with type 1 DM. In the absence of exercise, the most common precipitating factors for these conditions include inappropriate/inadequate insulin administration or infection.[10] In addition to the heightened risk due to lack of insulin as described here, the diabetic athlete is prone to elevated serum glucose levels and/or ketone production for several other reasons. Exercise alone, especially in athletes with baseline poor glucose control or elevated levels before activity, can cause an additional increase in serum glucose. Since insulin is not available to promote glucose uptake peripherally, the body responds by releasing counter-regulatory hormones, which cause an even greater rise in serum glucose levels.[5] At levels of extreme intensity, even in well-controlled diabetics, rising serum catecholamines exaggerate this response as well as promote free fatty acid and ketone body production, which can lead to DKA.[8] Under most circumstances, this is a transient response, and within 1 hour, hormone levels and serum glucose return to normal. In poorly controlled diabetic athletes, however, this response is prolonged, and individuals remain in a hyperglycemic state for extended periods of time, which may predispose them to ketoacidosis. Finally, the anticipatory stress of athletic competition, even before activity begins, causes a rise in counter-regulatory hormone release, leading to elevated blood glucose before physical activity, thus predisposing to hyperglycemia and ketosis.[8]

DKA is the most severe acute complication of hyperglycemia. DKA represents the body's response to cellular starvation in the setting of insulin deficiency and counter-regulatory (primarily glucagon) hormone excess[10] (**Fig. 1**). Under normal circumstances, insulin is responsible for the metabolism and storage of carbohydrates, fat, and protein. It exerts its actions on 3 major organs: liver, adipose tissue, and skeletal muscle. In the liver, insulin causes glucose uptake and conversion to glycogen stores, while inhibiting glycogen breakdown. In adipose tissue, insulin stimulates triglyceride production from free fatty acids and glycerol, and inhibits their breakdown. In skeletal muscle, it promotes the incorporation of amino acids into protein, while preventing amino acid release from both muscle and hepatic protein sources.[10]

In an insulin-deficient state, the body is unable to use glucose as fuel despite an elevated intravascular glucose level. The body responds by secreting counter-regulatory hormones (glucagon, catecholamines, cortisol, and growth hormone), precipitating a catabolic state. This leads to the breakdown of both protein and adipose stores as a potential source of intracellular fuel. Released free fatty acids are transported to the liver and converted to ketone bodies, primarily β-hydroxybutyric acid and acetoacetic acid. This process is further exaggerated in the setting of decreased hepatic glycogen stores. Without insulin, the body is unable to use these formed ketone bodies as an energy source. The end result is hyperglycemia, osmotic diuresis, and worsening ketonemia, leading to an anion-gap metabolic acidosis and DKA.[10]

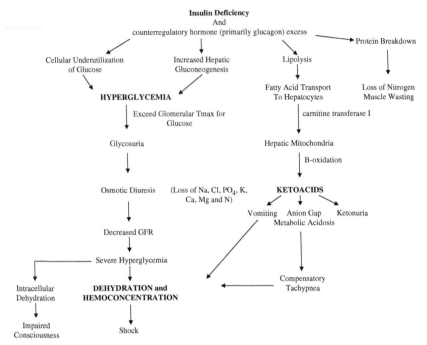

Fig. 1. Pathogenesis of DKA secondary to relative insulin deficiency and counter-regulatory hormone excess. (*From* Chansky ME, Lubkin CL. Diabetic ketoacidosis. In: Tintinalli JE, Kelen GD, Stapczynski JS, et al, editors. Emergency medicine: a comprehensive study guide. 6th edition. New York: McGraw-Hill; 2004. p. 1287; with permission.)

CLINICAL FEATURES

The classic clinical presentation of a patient in DKA includes a history of polydipsia, polyuria, dehydration, weight loss, generalized weakness, nausea/vomiting, and abdominal pain. Physical findings can include any of the following: tachycardia, hypotension, Kussmaul respirations (deep, rapid respirations), fruity odor on breath (secondary to acetone formation), poor skin turgor, altered mental status, and hypothermia.[11] These clinical manifestations are related to the primary metabolic derangements caused by hyperglycemia, volume depletion, and metabolic acidosis.[10] Hyperglycemia leads to an osmotic diuresis and volume loss, as well as profound renal-mediated electrolyte losses of sodium, potassium, chloride, phosphorous, calcium, and magnesium. In the early stages of the disease, patients may increase their fluid intake to compensate for these losses. However, as acidemia and ketosis progress, prostaglandins are released, causing peripheral vasodilation. Nausea and vomiting also occur, most likely as a maladaptive response to diminish acid load. Both responses, combined with continued diuresis, only contribute to a further state of overall volume and total body potassium depletion.[11]

Laboratory findings in DKA typically consist of the triad of hyperglycemia, ketonemia, and metabolic acidosis, combined with varying electrolyte abnormalities.[10] Patients usually present with serum glucose levels greater than 300 mg/dL, although lower initial levels may be seen in self-well-hydrated patients. Accumulation of ketoacids leads to acidemia and ketonuria, and the resultant anion-gap metabolic acidosis. The anion gap is calculated by subtracting the sum of the serum bicarbonate and chloride concentration from the measured serum sodium concentration [Na+ - (Cl⁻ + HCO3⁻)], with 6 to 12 mEq/L considered normal.[10] An elevated anion gap may be the only clue to the presence of an underlying metabolic acidosis, and cannot be overlooked.[11] Patients may also present with various electrolyte derangements. Patients typically present with pseudohyponatremia (caused by hyperglycemia and hyperlipidemia), and serum concentrations of potassium, magnesium, and phosphate may not accurately reflect the degree of total body deficit.[11] Serum sodium is typically depressed 2.4 mEq/dL for every 100 mg/dL elevation of serum glucose over 100 mg/dL, particularly with serum glucose levels greater than 400 mg/dL.[12]

TREATMENT

Because of the potential lethality and complications of untreated DKA, any athlete suspected to have DKA must be transported and treated in an emergency department setting. Patients should be placed on a monitor during transport and have at least one large-bore (16–18 gauge) intravenous line of normal saline (NS) running, as aggressive fluid therapy is the cornerstone of treatment.[10] Once in the hospital setting, a rapid bedside glucose determination, a urine dip for ketones, and an electrocardiogram should be performed. A venous blood gas should also be considered in critically ill patients, to quickly obtain pH (approximately 0.03 lower than arterial pH), pCO₂, and important electrolyte levels, specifically potassium. In addition, a complete blood count, chemistry panel (including magnesium, phosphate, and calcium and determination of anion gap), and urinalysis should be obtained[10] (**Fig. 2**). The goals of therapy include safe hydration and volume repletion along with correcting total body potassium deficiencies, metabolic acidosis, hyperglycemia, and other electrolyte disturbances at the approximate rate of occurrence. Meeting these goals safely involves carefully monitoring vital signs, electrolytes, anion gap, volume input/output, and insulin requirements until recovery is established.[11] It should be noted that correction of hyperglycemia alone is NOT the end point of treatment, as normalization of the anion gap indicates resolution of the metabolic acidosis in DKA.[10] The precipitating etiology of DKA should also be explored, including searching for an infectious source if indicated.

As stated above, rapid administration of intravenous fluids is the most critical step in the initial treatment of DKA. Hydration with isotonic saline will help to restore vital organ perfusion and improve renal clearance of glucose.[13] Fluid deficit in affected adult patients averages between 5 and 10 L. The choice of fluid replacement has not been well established, but it is generally recommended to begin with NS, which may prevent a rapid fall in extracellular osmolarity and thus a transfer of free water into the central nervous system, one theoretical etiology of cerebral edema.[10] After initial fluid replacement has begun, alternating with 0.5 NS or using 2 separate intravenous lines with normal and 0.5 NS has been advocated. A guideline for the rate of fluid replacement is 2 L within the first 2 hours, 2 L within the next 4 hours, and then 2 L in hours 6 through 12.[10] Intravenous fluids should be changed to D5 0.5 NS once blood glucose levels approach 300 mg/dL, to prevent hypoglycemia.[10] Although beyond the scope of this review, the particularly young athlete with new-onset diabetes and DKA may be at increased risk for cerebral edema, and fluid management should be adjusted according to pediatric critical care guidelines.

Supplemental insulin can be administered once initial laboratory data have returned, specifically determination of serum potassium concentration. On presentation, the vast majority of patients have initial potassium levels greater than 3.3 mEq/dL, secondary to acidosis and volume depletion, despite profound total body deficits.

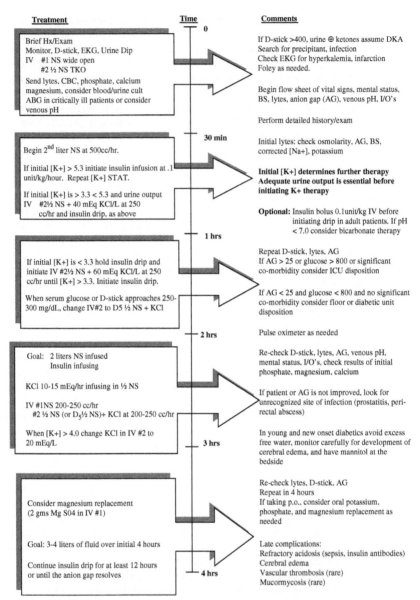

Treatment	Time	Comments
Brief Hx/Exam Monitor, D-stick, EKG, Urine Dip IV #1 NS wide open #2 ½ NS TKO Send lytes, CBC, phosphate, calcium magnesium, consider blood/urine cult ABG in critically ill patients or consider venous pH	0	If D-stick >400, urine ⊕ ketones assume DKA Search for precipitant, infection Check EKG for hyperkalemia, infarction Foley as needed. Begin flow sheet of vital signs, mental status, BS, lytes, anion gap (AG), venous pH, I/O's Perform detailed history/exam
Begin 2nd liter NS at 500cc/hr. If initial [K+] > 5.3 initiate insulin infusion at .1 unit/kg/hour. Repeat [K+] STAT. If initial [K+] is > 3.3 < 5.3 and urine output IV #2½ NS + 40 mEq KCl/L at 250 cc/hr and insulin drip, as above	30 min	Initial lytes: check osmolarity, AG, BS, corrected [Na+], potassium **Initial [K+] determines further therapy Adequate urine output is essential before initiating K+ therapy** **Optional:** Insulin bolus 0.1unit/kg IV before initiating drip in adult patients. If pH < 7.0 consider bicarbonate therapy
If initial [K+] is < 3.3 hold insulin drip and initiate IV #2½ NS + 60 mEq KCl/L at 250 cc/hr until [K+] > 3.3. Initiate insulin drip. When serum glucose or D-stick approaches 250- 300 mg/dL, change IV#2 to D5 ½ NS + KCl	1 hrs	Repeat D-stick, lytes, AG If AG > 25 or glucose > 800 or significant co-morbidity consider ICU disposition If AG < 25 and glucose < 800 and no significant co-morbidity consider floor or diabetic unit disposition Pulse oximeter as needed
Goal: 2 liters NS infused Insulin infusing KCl 10-15 mEq/hr infusing in ½ NS IV #1NS 200-250 cc/hr #2 ½ NS (or D5½ NS)+ KCl at 200-250 cc/hr When [K+] > 4.0 change KCl in IV #2 to 20 mEq/L	2 hrs 3 hrs	Re-check D-stick, lytes, AG, venous pH, mental status, I/O's, check results of initial phosphate, magnesium, calcium If patient or AG is not improved, look for unrecognized site of infection (prostatitis, peri- rectal abscess) In young and new onset diabetics avoid excess free water, monitor carefully for development of cerebral edema, and have mannitol at the bedside
Consider magnesium replacement (2 gms Mg S04 in IV #1) Goal: 3-4 liters of fluid over initial 4 hours Continue insulin drip for at least 12 hours or until the anion gap resolves	4 hrs	Re-check lytes, D-stick, AG Repeat in 4 hours If taking p.o., consider oral potassium, phosphate, and magnesium replacement as needed Late complications: Refractory acidosis (sepsis, insulin antibodies) Cerebral edema Vascular thrombosis (rare) Mucormycosis (rare)

Fig. 2. Timeline for the typical patient with suspected DKA. (*Adapted from* Chansky ME, Lubkin CL. Diabetic ketoacidosis. In: Tintinalli J, Kelen GD, Stapczynski JS, et al, editors. Emergency medicine: a comprehensive study guide. 6th edition. New York: McGraw-Hill; 2004. p. 1290; with permission.)

The potential danger of initiating insulin therapy with low initial serum potassium is an intracellular shift, resulting in profound hypokalemia. If initial potassium is below 3.3 mEq/dL, insulin should be held, and an oral dose of 40 mEq of potassium should be given 15 to 30 minutes before insulin therapy or documentation of serum potassium concentration greater than 3.3 mEq/dL.[13] Intravenous potassium supplementation (10–15 mEq/h in a monitored setting) should be reserved for the vomiting patient.

Potassium levels between 3.3 and 5.0 mEq/dL should prompt a minimum of 10 mEq/h replacement intravenously, in addition to simultaneous insulin therapy.[10] Potassium levels greater than 5.0 mEq/dL should prompt insulin therapy alone, with careful attention to hourly monitoring of potassium, as therapy with fluids and insulin will predictably lower serum potassium concentration acutely.[10]

Insulin replacement should be in a controlled manner as a continuous infusion, as boluses are thought to be less physiologic and no longer accepted as standard, especially in children and adolescents. The initial infusion dose should be 0.1 U/kg/h.[10] Subcutaneous and intramuscular injections are not recommended, as absorption will be erratic in an ill and volume-depleted patient.[14] A poor response to initial infusion rates should lead to increasing dosages by doubling the infusion rate.[13] Therapy should be continued until the anion gap has closed. A common method of objective disease progression is to check hourly finger stick glucose and every other hourly serum chemistries.[10]

Careful attention must be paid to other electrolytes such as phosphate, magnesium, and bicarbonate. Phosphate should be replaced as needed and done so via oral route, unless severe or symptomatic (rare) hypophosphatemia (below 1.0 mg/dL) is present. Failure to replenish phosphate can rarely lead to hypoxia, rhabdomyolysis, hemolysis, respiratory failure, and cardiac dysfunction.[14] Complications of hypomagnesemia are also rare, and magnesium replacement can generally be accomplished by oral replacement.[10] Finally, bicarbonate therapy is a controversial issue and is not routinely recommended.[15] Advocates argue that therapy may improve myocardial contractility, elevate ventricular fibrillation threshold, improve catecholamine tissue response, and decrease work of breathing.[16] The disadvantages may include, but are not limited to, worsening hypokalemia, paradoxic central nervous system acidosis and intracellular acidosis, sodium overload, and precipitation of cerebral edema.[17] To date not a single randomized study has demonstrated any benefit to the administration of bicarbonate in DKA, and patients routinely recover from a very low initial pH with appropriate therapy.[10]

The vast majority of athletes presenting with DKA are admitted to a monitored bed with experience handling continuous insulin infusions or a critical care setting. A minority of patients with mild forms of the disease (anion gap less than 18 mEq/L, glucose less than 300 mg/dL) may be managed in the emergency department for several hours and discharged with appropriate close follow-up.[10]

PREVENTION PLAN

The most effective strategy of the discussed diabetic emergencies is prevention. Prevention strategy is multidisciplinary and involves educating the patient, parents, athletic trainers, and primary care doctor and involving an endocrinologist. Pillars of avoiding disaster include having a preparticipation physical examination, diabetes care plan, recognition education, and treatment education.

Preparticipation physical examination should assess hemoglobin A_{1c} (HbA$_{1c}$) quarterly to gain a general idea of the patient's diabetic management. HbA$_{1c}$ of 7% or less is recommended by the American Diabetic Association for adults and of less than 7.5% for teens and adolescents, with 7% correlating with an average blood glucose level of approximately 150 mg/dL. The American Association of Clinical Endocrinologists has tighter recommendations for glycemic control, and individual goals should be discussed with the patient's medical team.[18] These levels serve as an overall measurement of an individual's glycemic control over a 3-month period and not day-to-day variations.

Other aspects of the pre-participation physical examination in a young diabetic should include ophthalmologic examinations annually beginning 3 to 5 years after diagnosis, to screen for retinopathy, glaucoma, and cataracts. Diabetic nephropathy screening should take place 5 years after diagnosis by urine analysis for protein, and neuropathy screening, 5 years after diagnosis is made and annually thereafter.[18] Neuropathy may affect tactile sensation and reflexes and be especially important in weight-bearing athletes, those with tight shoes, frequent blisters, or who walk barefoot. Less recognized effects of diabetic neuropathy include autonomic neuropathy, which may blunt the patient's ability to recognize hypoglycemia or cause exercise intolerance or orthostatic hypotension. Finally, cardiovascular examination including exercise stress test should be performed after 15 years or sooner for those with additional cardiovascular risk factors.[18]

Diabetic care plans may be the cornerstone of effective deterrence of DKA. Patients should be educated and motivated for frequent blood glucose monitoring. This should be done 2 to 3 times at 30-minute intervals before exercise to trend direction of blood glucose levels and thereafter every 30 minutes during exercise. Additional monitoring should be done every 2 hours for up to 4 hours postexertion to monitor for delayed hypoglycemia. For those participating in sports late at night, monitoring should occur at minimum directly before sleep and immediately upon waking, with some recommending one time monitoring during the night.[8]

Predetermined blood glucose levels should be set with the patient's physician and athletic trainer for barring participation from play. Generally, if the pre-exercise level is less than 100 mg/dL, carbohydrate supplementation should take place. If levels are over 180 mg/dL, the athlete should consume a noncarbohydrate containing fluid to prevent dehydration.[8]

There is a multitude of specific issues regarding insulin use and monitoring in the athlete, and detailed knowledge will help prevent medication misuse and over- or undertreatment before participation. Administration should be subcutaneous and not intramuscular, as the intramuscular route may lead to fast absorption and high insulin peaks during activity. This can be attributed to increased blood flow to the musculature during sport participation as well as the effect of heat on absorption rates. Care must be taken in extreme heat environments, sauna, whirlpool, and hot shower after injection. Cold will have opposing effects on absorption, so ice packs and other cold exposure should similarly be avoided.[8]

Athletes with insulin pumps should change infusion sets 2 to 3 times weekly to avoid skin and infusion site irritation. It also must be recognized that extreme temperatures, generally below freezing or above 86 degrees F, can reduce insulin activity.[8] Therefore, this type of exposure should prompt replacement of the insulin-filled cartridge and infusion set. Other issues to consider with insulin pump therapy include damage during contact sports, disconnection during vigorous movements, and infusion set displacement from excessive sweating by deactivating the pump adhesive.

The diabetic patient must carefully make his or her travel preparations in conjunction with the health care team and athletic trainer. A diabetic patient is allowed to travel on an airplane with carefully labeled diabetic supplies. A travel kit should include unused syringes, blood glucose meters, test strips, lancets, alcohol swabs, insulin, insulin pump if needed and supplies, glucagon emergency kit, and ketone testing supplies. The athlete should generally have at least 2 times as much medication and testing equipment that is thought to be needed. Supplies should be carried with the person at all times and not stowed underneath an airplane. Additionally, extra prescriptions for these supplies should be carried with the athlete as a precaution. Prepackaged meals or snacks should be available, especially if food will not be available for any period of time. A letter from the athlete's physician stating the medical condition and necessity of supplies as well as health insurance card and emergency contact numbers should be included in the travel kit. An identification card stating medical condition of diabetes may also be helpful, and, finally, if traveling abroad, it is advisable to learn basic phrases that will alert natives that the patient has diabetes or needs sugar, water, insulin, or health care.[8]

SUMMARY

DM is a chronic endocrine disorder affecting many children, adolescents, and young adults participating in athletics. If not properly managed, diabetes can lead to many serious complications during exercise, including hypoglycemia, hyperglycemia, and potentially lethal DKA. All individuals directly involved in the care of a diabetic athlete should be aware of the clinical signs and symptoms of hyperglycemia and DKA, and if suspected, patients should be transported to the nearest hospital monitored, with an NS infusion, and treated according to recommended guidelines. It is crucial that all diabetic athletes work with their families, physician, and trainers to create individualized plans of treatment according to the level of activity and severity of disease, as education and prevention are paramount in avoiding most severe complications.

REFERENCES

1. Inzucchi S, Porte D, Sherwin R, et al. The classification and diagnosis of diabetes mellitus. In: The diabetes mellitus manual. New York: McGraw-Hill; 2005.
2. CDC's Diabetes program publications and products: national diabetes fact sheet 2007. Available at: http://www.cdc.gov/diabetes/pubs/estimates07.htm. Accessed September 8, 2008.
3. Bennet PH, Knowler WC. Definition diagnosis and classification of diabetes mellitus and impaired glucose tolerance. In: Kahn CR, Weir GC, King GL, editors. Joslin's diabetes mellitus. 14th edition. Philadelphia: Lippincott Williams & Wilkins; 2004. p. 331–41.
4. Rush M, Winslett S, Wisdom KD. Diabetes mellitus. In: Tintinalli J, Kelen GD, Stapczynski JS, editors. Emergency medicine: a comprehensive study guide. 6th edition. New York: McGraw-Hill; 2004. p. 1294–304.
5. Jimenez CC. Diabetes and exercise: the role of the athletic trainer. J Athl Train 1997;32(4):339–43.
6. Lisle DK, Trojian TH. Managing the athlete with Type I diabetes. Curr Sports Med Rep 2006;5:93–8.
7. Hough DO. Diabetes mellitus in sports. Med Clin North Am 1988;72:1301–21.
8. Jimenez CC, Corcoran MH, Crawley JT, et al. National athletic trainers' association position statement: management of the athlete with Type I diabetes mellitus. J Athl Train 2007;42(4):536–45.
9. Wasserman DH, Zinman B. Exercise in individuals with insulin dependent diabetes mellitus. Diabetes Care 1994;17:924–37.
10. Chansky ME, Lubkin CL. Diabetic ketoacidosis. In: Tintinalli J, Kelen GD, Stapczynski JS, editors. Emergency medicine: a comprehensive study guide. 6th edition. New York: McGraw-Hill; 2004. p. 1287–94.
11. Kitabchi A, Kreisberg R, Murphy MB, et al. Hyperglycemic crises in adult patients with diabetes: a consensus statement from the American Diabetes Association. Diabetes Care 2006;29(12):2739–48.
12. Hillier TA, Abbott RD, Barrett EJ. Hyponatremia: evaluating the correction factor for hyperglycemia. Am J Med 1999;106:399–403.

13. American Diabetes Association. Clinical practice recommendations. Diabetes Care 2002;25(suppl 1):S100–8.
14. Foster DW, McGarry JD. The metabolic derangements and treatment of diabetic ketoacidosis. N Engl J Med 1983;309:159–69.
15. Lebovitz HE. Diabetic ketoacidosis. Lancet 1995;345:767–72.
16. Green SM, Rothrock SG, Ho JD, et al. Failure of adjunctive bicarbonate to improve outcome in severe pediatric diabetic ketoacidosis. Emerg Med 1998; 31:41–8.
17. Okuda Y, Adrogue HJ, Field JB, et al. Does bicarbonate therapy improve the management of severe diabetic ketoacidosis. J Clin Endocrinol Metab 1996;81: 314–20.
18. American Diabetes Association. Position statement: physical activity/exercise and diabetes mellitus. Diabetes Care 2003;26(Suppl):S73–7.

The Daily Management of Athletes with Diabetes

John M. MacKnight, MD[a,b], Dilaawar J. Mistry, MD, MS, ATC[a,*],
Joyce Green Pastors, RD, MS, CDE[c], Viola Holmes, RD, MS[d],
Corey A. Rynders, BA[e]

KEYWORDS

- Diabetes • Exercise • Nutrition • Management • Insulin
- Complications

Competitive athletes with diabetes present a significant challenge to themselves and the medical staff who care for them on a daily basis. The physiological demands induced by intense exercise and training, nutritional needs and varied meal timing to support and enhance training regimens and competition, and the stress of competition are just a few factors that athletes with diabetes endure during their daily management.

They are also at risk for both acute hypoglycemia or ketoacidosis and chronic complications—microvascular and macrovascular disease. Therefore, a thorough understanding of the unique metabolic demands is critical to their systematic, thorough management. This article provides a general overview of exercise and nutritional considerations and a detailed review of the management of diabetic athletes.

THE DIABETIC ATHLETE—EXERCISE CONSIDERATIONS
Diabetes and Exercise—An Overview

Athletic participation is considered safe for individuals with diabetes mellitus (DM) and is typically recommended as part of "long-term" treatment plans.[1–3]

Nevertheless, because many sports place unpredictable energy demands on the athlete with diabetes, it is imperative that these individuals work closely with their

[a] Department of Internal Medicine, UVA Sports Medicine, University of Virginia Health System, P.O. Box 801004, 545 Ray C. Hunt #240m Charlottesville, VA 22908, USA
[b] Department of Orthopaedic Surgery, UVA Sports Medicine, University of Virginia Health System, Charlottesville, VA 22908, USA
[c] Virginia Center for Diabetes, Professional Education, Department of Medicine/Division of Endocrinology, University of Virginia Health System, Box 801417, Charlottesville, VA, USA
[d] Diabetes Education and Management Program, Department of Nutrition Services, University of Virginia Health System, PO Box 800873, Charlottesville, VA, USA
[e] Department of Human Services, University of Virginia, PO Box 400407, Memorial Gymnasium, 210 Emmet Street, Charlottesville, VA 22903, USA
* Corresponding author.
E-mail address: dm5f@virginia.edu (D.J. Mistry).

Clin Sports Med 28 (2009) 479–495
doi:10.1016/j.csm.2009.02.005
0278-5919/09/$ – see front matter
sportsmed.theclinics.com

physicians, trainers, and coaches to develop effective pre-exercise management plans to avoid the harmful consequences associated with poor glycemic control.

The American Diabetes Association (ADA) has classified DM into 2 general forms; type 1 diabetes (T1D) and type 2 diabetes (T2D). There are an estimated 16 million people living in the United States with DM, of whom 10% have T1D and 80% to 90% have T2D. The prevalence of T2D, which is highest among African Americans, is increasing at an alarming rate both in the United States of America and worldwide.[4] Unfortunately, the incidence of this disease is also increasing among children and adolescents.[5]

T1D results from a highly specific immune-mediated destruction of pancreatic β cells, leading to chronic hyperglycemia. Individuals with T1D are usually diagnosed in adolescence and must rely on the injection of exogenous insulin for survival.[6] Interestingly, in 1950, a diagnosis of T1D was associated with a 1 in 5 risk of mortality within 10 years.[7] However, due to several advances in insulin therapy and methods for self–blood glucose monitoring, individuals with T1D now live near-normal life spans and are capable of competing at the highest levels of sport (eg, Olympic games) and in the most extreme endurance events (eg, Ironman triathlon). Yet effective management is a constant challenge, because insulin therapy is an "imperfect science."

Conversely, T2D correlates strongly with obesity and unhealthy lifestyle behaviors (poor diet, smoking, physical inactivity, etc), and diagnosis is often delayed.[8] The hallmark characteristic of T2D is insulin resistance, which is characterized by a defect in the ability of skeletal muscle to respond to insulin-mediated glucose uptake.[6] Additionally, with advancing disease, pancreatic β-cell dysfunction results in increasingly less insulin secretion.[8]

Although regular exercise is generally thought to be most beneficial in the long-term management of T2D, it is rare to encounter young, competitive athletes with T2D. This is because most individuals are usually diagnosed with the T2D later in adulthood (∼age 40 years), yet, alarmingly maintain sedentary lifestyles.[1] However, with an increasing emphasis being placed on the importance of physical activity, it is probable that a greater percentage of individuals with T2D will participate in recreational sports as "masters" athletes.

T2D is also rapidly increasing at an alarming rate in adolescents.[5] Early therapeutic intervention is imperative, and their teachers and parents should encourage participation in physical activity, which may positively influence compliance with exercise programs in adulthood. Children with T2D may participate in sports as part of their usual school curriculum or may be motivated by external factors, such as the desire to "fit-in" socially.

This section first reviews substrate regulation during moderate- and high-intensity exercise under normal circumstances. Subsequently, exercise considerations in athletes with T1D and T2D are discussed. A majority of the discussion in this section focuses on exercise considerations in individuals with T1D, since it is more prevalent in competitive athletes; however, implications of exercise in T2D are also reviewed.

Overview of Normal Glucoregulation During Exercise

Metabolic responses to exercise are determined primarily by the intensity (ie, moderate or intense), duration (ie, short, prolonged, or intermittent), and environmental conditions (ie, hot, humid, time of day). During moderate-intensity exercise (40%–59% of maximal oxygen consumption [Vo_2 max] or 55%–69% of maximum heart rate), the fuel for muscular contraction is obtained almost exclusively from aerobic metabolism—by using a mixture of carbohydrate (CHO) from muscle glycogen stores and circulating free fatty acids (FFA) as fuel. Most endurance sports are performed within the moderate-intensity domain (eg, long-distance running and cycling).

The transition from rest to moderate-intensity exercise is characterized by an increase in sympathetic nervous activity, which aids in increasing endogenous glucose production by the liver (gluconeogenesis) and stimulates the release of FFA from adipose tissue (lipolysis). In addition, α-adrenergic stimulation of pancreatic islet cells inhibits insulin secretion, which in turn signals the release of glucagon from pancreatic α cells. Since high insulin levels normally inhibit glycogenolysis and hepatic gluconeogenesis, a decrease in insulin effectively primes the liver to the effects of glucagon. This mechanism precisely matches glucose utilization by exercising muscle tissue for hepatic glucose production and is the key factor maintaining blood glucose within a narrow range during moderate-intensity exercise (80–100 mg/dL).[9] The decrease in insulin is a critical mechanism to balance glucose utilization at the muscle, which may reach ~3 mg/kg/min, and prevent hypoglycemia and maintain the ability to exercise effectively.[10]

It is important to note that hepatic sources of glucose, derived from liver glycogen stores or produced via gluconeogenesis, are able to enter muscle cells despite low insulin concentrations for mainly 2 reasons: (1) exercise independently increases glucose transport via a pathway independent of insulin-stimulated glucose uptake,[11] and (2) muscle contraction results in the enhanced recruitment of capillaries, which augments the surface area available for nutrient exchange.[12] It is well known that muscle contraction increases glucose transport even in the complete absence of insulin[13] and that the synergistic effects of insulin and muscle contraction are additive to enhanced glucose transport.[14] Sustained muscular contraction during exercise also provides an improvement in insulin sensitivity, which may extend for several hours, lasting into the postexercise period.[15]

High-intensity exercise, 85% to 100% Vo_2 max or greater than 90% maximal heart rate, sustained for 10 to 30 minutes or intermittent bouts of 3 to 5 minutes is common in team-oriented sports, such as lacrosse, football, hockey, soccer, track and field, and swimming. Exercise to Vo_2 max is sustained primarily by aerobic metabolism, including oxidative phosphorylation and to a limited extent, beta oxidation. In contrast, high-intensity, supramaximal-effort (>Vo_2 max) activities sustained for only 3 to 30 seconds use the anaerobic energy system (glycolysis and the Adenosine triphosphate-phosphocreatine [ATP-PCr system]). In either situation, high-intensity exercise is highly dependent on glucose as a fuel, derived from either hepatic or muscle glycogenolysis. In addition, exercise at high intensity is characterized by lactate accumulation and a marked increase in catecholamine (norepinephrine and epinephrine) concentrations, by up to 14- to 18-folds above basal levels. This is in sharp contrast to moderate-intensity exercise in which catecholamine levels increase by only 2- to 4-folds above baseline.[9]

During high-intensity exercise, hepatic glucose production exceeds muscle glucose utilization, resulting in slight hyperglycemia. This is largely due to the fact that norepinephrine and, to a lesser extent, epinephrine act as powerful stimulators of muscle and liver glycogenolysis. Norepinephrine reaches the liver as a "spillover" from other tissues or by direct sympathetic nerve stimulation, which results in increased hepatic glucose production. Moreover, akin to moderate-intensity exercise, insulin levels remain very close to basal levels despite the fact that glucose production exceeds utilization.[9]

In the immediate postexercise period, insulin levels rapidly increase both in response to high blood glucose levels and following removal of circulating catecholamines. The next 20 to 60 minutes are characterized by a state of hyperglycemia and hyperinsulinemia, which creates an environment favorable for glycogen replenishment in anticipation of future exercise.[9]

Exercise Considerations in Athletes with Type 1 Diabetes

Compared to healthy peers, athletes with T1D experience nearly all the same health-related benefits from exercise.[2] These include improvements in health-related quality of life, reduction in blood pressure, improvement in lipid abnormalities (ie, high low-density lipoprotein cholesterol, triglycerides),[16] increased insulin sensitivity, decreased insulin requirements, lower hemoglobin A_{1c} (HbA_{1c}) levels,[17] improved endothelial function,[18] and improvement in cardiorespiratory fitness (Vo_2 max), which has repeatedly been shown to be a powerful predictor of future cardiovascular disease (CVD).[19]

Despite these benefits, without proper, proactive education and precautions, exercise may predispose the diabetic athlete to hypoglycemia—the most common adverse event associated with insulin therapy.[10] For good reasons, individuals with T1D should be encouraged to maintain "tight" glucose control to lower HbA_{1c} levels to a measure that strongly correlates with a lower risk of long-term complications, including peripheral neuropathy, retinopathy, nephropathy, and CVD. It is important to note, however, that the Diabetes Complications and Controls Trial (DCCT) reported a significant 3-fold increase in the incidence of hypoglycemia in individuals with strict glycemic control on insulin therapy.[20] In addition, it is hard to simulate "precompetition" anxiety and excitement, which tends to increase blood glucose above and beyond levels noted and treated during "practice". Finally, exercise in hot and humid environments can increase counter-regulatory responses to high-intensity exercise as well as alter the rate of insulin absorption.[21] Thus, athletes with T1D need to find a suitable balance with their exercise regimens, nutritional adequacy, and insulin dosing to avoid either hypo- or hyperglycemia.

Exercise Considerations in Athletes with Type 2 Diabetes

Exercise training in T2D results in increased translocation of muscle glucose transporter-4 receptors, an increased capacity for insulin-stimulated glucose uptake, and decreased insulin resistance. The defects in insulin signaling and/or secretion cannot be fully reversed, yet increased physical activity as a routine "lifestyle" change is a major intervention in the management of T2D.[1]

To further highlight the importance of "lifestyle" change in the treatment of T2D, the Diabetes Prevention Program (DPP) trial concluded in 2002 that after ~3 years, "lifestyle" interventions reduced the incidence of diabetes by 58% compared with only 31% in a group treated with the antidiabetic drug metformin.[22] Currently, the ADA recommends that all individuals with T2D engage in at least 150 min/wk of moderate to vigorous-intensity exercise.[3]

Other important exercise considerations in T2D, especially in those being treated for concomitant hypertension, include the potential for negative electrolyte homeostasis (diuretics), reduction of exercise capacity and athletic performance during high-intensity exercise (β-blockers), and increased susceptibility to hypoglycemia (aspirin or angiotensin-converting enzyme [ACE] inhibitors). The mechanisms by which aspirin or ACE inhibitors may induce hypoglycemia is poorly understood.[3]

Unfortunately, the majority of individuals with T2D are not likely to engage in physical activity,[1] yet the benefits of exercise far outweigh risks of either hypoglycemia or hyperglycemia and should be a major component of any therapeutic intervention.

THE DIABETIC ATHLETE—NUTRITIONAL CONSIDERATIONS
Healthy Eating for Peak Performance—Balance of Nutrients

In order to exercise and compete at peak levels of performance, diabetic athletes have unique nutritional needs. Optimal blood glucose management to prevent hypo- or hyperglycemia is a daunting task and requires a thorough understanding of the current recommendations for caloric and fluid intake before, during, and after exercise. In addition to balanced and timely CHO intake, diabetic diets should contain optimal amounts of proteins and fats that provide calories and have essential functions for glycemic control and health.

The recommended balance of these energy-yielding nutrients for athletes does not differ significantly from recommendations for the general population. However, additional calories and fluids may be required for diabetic athletes and depends upon exercise intensity, total energy expenditure, type of exercise and training program, duration of exercise, gender, and environmental circumstances. Calorie requirements can range from 2,000 to more than 6,000 cal/d. Therefore, a thorough nutritional assessment of "usual" food intake followed by monitoring of weight, appetite, and blood glucose levels is the best way to evaluate adequacy of caloric intake.[23]

A joint position statement by the ADA, Dietitians for Canada, and the American College of Sports Medicine has recommended the following general energy requirements for competitive athletes.[24]

1. CHO consumption range of 6 to 10 g/kg body weight is required to maintain blood glucose levels during and after exercise and for replacement of glycogen stores.
2. Protein consumption range of 1.2 to 1.7 g/kg body weight. Generally, this level of protein can be obtained from the diet. Protein is needed for tissue repair and muscle growth.
   a. For endurance athletes, 1.2 to 1.4 g/kg body weight.
   b. For strength-trained athletes, 1.6 to 1.7 g/kg body weight.
3. Fat consumption range of 20% to 25% of total daily calories. Fat provides needed calories as well as fat-soluble vitamins, and essential fatty acids. No performance benefits have been found in reducing fat intake to less than 15% of daily calories.

Healthy Eating for Peak Performance—Timing and Types of Nutrients

Diabetic athletes who participate in regular endurance exercise should consume ~60% CHO daily[23] and coordinate food intake with "timing" of exercise and insulin dosing. This approach is critical for optimal glycemic control, to maintain muscle and liver glycogen stores, prevent fatigue, optimize exercise performance, and prevent complications.

Carbohydrate intake before exercise
General principles and recommendations for timing and choices for food include the following:

1. Eating an easily digested meal in the amount of 200 to 350 g (or 4 g/kg of body weight) of CHO 3 to 6 hours before an exercise event has been shown to enhance performance.[25,26]
2. Although 60 to 90 g of CHO are recommended per meal in most adults with diabetes, athletes with diabetes who "CHO load" (200–350 g per meal) to increase glycogen stores before long athletic events[27] should monitor blood glucose levels regularly and adjust insulin doses accordingly.

3. The recommended pre-event CHO intake is approximately 1 g of CHO/kg of body weight 1 hour before the exercise. Low-fat CHO foods, such as crackers, muffins, toast, fruit, and yogurt, instead of sugary sweets are good choices.
4. If the exercise is of short duration (<45 minutes), a pre-exercise snack of ~15 g of CHO eaten 15 to 30 minutes before the event has been reported to be an adequate amount.[28]
5. Foods such as pancakes, potatoes, bread, and fruit are appropriate choices.

Carbohydrate intake during exercise

CHO are needed during exercise of long duration to maintain CHO oxidation and to replenish muscle glycogen stores on a regular basis.[29] As stated previously, the recommended percentage CHO consumption for an athlete with diabetes, either during training or an event, is ~60%, which equates to 6 to 10 g of CHO/kg body weight, depending on the duration of the exercise period. Because average CHO intake is generally 4 to 5 g/kg body weight per day (~45% of calories), increasing CHO may be an additional challenge for the exercising athlete.[23] Recommendations include[30] the following:

1. For exercise periods of 1 h/d, 5 to 6 g CHO/kg body weight.
2. For exercise periods more than 2 h/d, 8 g CHO/kg body weight may be needed.
3. For endurance activities, this may be increased to 10 g CHO/kg body weight.
4. During prolonged (>45–60 minutes) or intense exercise (>80% maximal heart rate), an intake of 15 g CHO every 30 to 60 minutes of activity is a safe starting guideline.[23]
5. Solid or liquid forms of CHO may be consumed. Each form has its distinct advantages. Liquids provide fluid for hydration, whereas solids may prevent hunger. For exercise lasting more than 60 to 90 minutes, a liquid CHO form is most recommended, because it is more practical and contributes to adequate hydration.[31]

Carbohydrate intake after exercise

1. Consuming CHO immediately after exercise as opposed to waiting for a period of time has been shown to replace CHO stores more efficiently.
2. Intake of 1.5 g of CHO/kg body weight within 30 minutes after an extended exercise session (lasting >90 minutes) and intake of an additional 1.5 g of CHO/kg body weight 1 to 2 hours later will replete glycogen to pre-exercise levels and will reduce risk of postexercise hypoglycemia.[32]
3. Blood glucose levels should be monitored at 1- or 2-hour intervals to assess the response to exercise and to make the necessary adjustments in insulin and food intake.

Adjustment of carbohydrate and insulin

A reduction in the dose of insulin before exercise may be required. A reduction of short-acting insulin of 30% to 50% has been reported to decrease the risk of hypoglycemia.[33] Another method is to decrease the insulin used during exercise by 10% of the total daily insulin dose.[23] This approach is discussed in more detail later in the article.

Hypoglycemia—nutritional prevention

In order to prevent the most common complication of exercise in diabetic athletes, the amount of CHO, fat, and protein consumed before, during, and after exercise should be determined by blood glucose levels and the proposed duration of exercise.

1. Planned pre-exercise snacks should be high in CHO, low in fat, and moderate in protein content.
2. The postexercise snack should consist of CHO and protein.

3. Examples of pre- or postexercise snack choices include the following:
   a. CHO: whole-grain bread, breadsticks, crackers, cereal, fig bars, oatmeal-raisin cookies, granola bar, fruit, juice, yogurt, and milk.
   b. Protein: 1 to 2 oz lean meat, nut butter, and cheese.
4. Diabetic athletes should also have fast-acting CHO sources readily available. Fifteen grams of CHO will raise blood glucose 30 to 50 points within a 15- to 30-minute timeframe.[34] Convenient fast-acting CHO sources include glucose gels, 3 to 4 glucose tablets, 2 tablespoons of raisins, 1/2 cup fruit juice, or 1 cup low-fat or nonfat milk.

Nutritional Myths

Athletes often believe that nutritional supplements improve performance. However, adequate consumption from a variety of food sources precludes the need for vitamin and mineral supplements. The 2005 Dietary Guidelines for Healthy Americans emphasize that supplements may be useful when they fill a specific identified "nutrient-gap" that either cannot or is not being met by an individual's intake of food. Nutrient supplements are not a substitute for a healthy diet.[35] In addition, any supplements or ergogenic aids being considered for use should be evaluated by a trained health care professional. Stringent regulations on the nutritional supplement industry are sparse; therefore, caution is advised on the use of supplements.

Consuming large amounts of protein and protein supplements is also a common practice of athletes. Studies have found that large amounts of protein (>2.4 g/kg/d) may place undue stress on the kidneys.[36] In the athlete with diabetes, this may compound the risk of long-term renal complications.

Fluids and Electrolytes

It is a well-established fact that the thirst mechanism is blunted with exercise.[37] Therefore, in order to prevent complications secondary to dehydration, diabetic athletes should monitor and consume adequate fluid before, during, and after exercise.[24] Adequate hydration helps prevent a rise in "core" body temperature and reduces heat-induced stress of the cardiovascular system. Cool, plain water is recommended as the beverage of choice.

Recommendations for fluid intake for persons with diabetes engaging in physical activity include 3 cups of water ~2 hours before an event. Another 1 to 2 cups of water should be consumed 10 to 15 minutes before the beginning of the event.[24] The most effective method to monitor fluid needs during exercise is to note weight changes from fluid losses during exercise. Approximately 2 cups of fluid should be consumed for every pound lost. Persons who are sedentary lose approximately a quart of water daily from sweating, whereas athletes undergoing strenuous exercise may lose more than or equal to 2 qt.[23] Specifically, during exercise, the athlete should continue drinking small amounts (1/2–1 cup) of fluid at 10- to 20-minute intervals. This is necessary to ensure replacement of body fluid lost by sweating and to maintain optimal blood volume. Furthermore, consumption of small amounts of fluids at frequent intervals can reduce abdominal discomfort and "bloating."

For exercise sessions greater than or equal to 60 minutes, beverages that contain at least 8% CHO (eg, sports drinks or diluted fruit juices of 50% dilution) are the best source of "replacement" beverages, because they replace fluid and calories.[23] Drinks with a concentration of sugars greater than 10%, via increased osmosis, can produce undesirable gastrointestinal symptoms, such as cramps, nausea, diarrhea, or bloating. Fruit juices and regular soft drinks contain about 12% CHO and should be diluted with an equal amount of water prior to consumption. Ounce for ounce, common sports drinks such as Gatorade and PowerADE contain less CHO than soft drinks or fruit juices and have a lower osmolality, which may make them more desirable for consumption during exercise.

Because individuals differ in their metabolic responses to exercise, dictated by varying levels of emotional and physical stress of competition, we recommend that in the postexercise period, rehydration be guided by estimation of body weight and blood glucose levels. Diabetics should work with their athletic trainers, nutritionists, and physicians to determine individualized needs for either plain water or an additional CHO-containing beverage to promote euhydration and normoglycemia.[23]

THE DIABETIC ATHLETE—MANAGEMENT
Education

Appropriate glucose management in diabetic athletes is dependent on both the athlete and the care provider having a firm understanding of the pathophysiology of diabetes and its nuances with respect to athletic participation. The cornerstone of management for T1D athletes is the prevention of both hypo- and hyperglycemia while maintaining adequate energy balance for exercise performance. Exercise for T1D is a nutritional challenge[38,39] because of the delicate balance between insulin use and caloric intake. In contrast, T2D should be viewed as an energy-excess syndrome in which skeletal muscles and the liver become progressively insulin resistant. As skeletal muscle accounts for the major site of insulin-stimulated glucose utilization in humans, endurance or combined endurance and resistance exercise training may improve overall glucose tolerance and/or insulin sensitivity[40,41] but may also create challenges in optimal glucose control.

All diabetic athletes should be educated about the importance of establishing a daily pattern of consistency for all aspects of their diabetes management. It is ideal to have the athlete begin a routine of insulin and/or oral medication administration, consistent caloric intake, regimented exercise program every day, and frequent monitoring of blood glucose levels. Each of these steps will not only aid in maximizing blood glucose control but also help the diabetic athlete understand how best to manage the diabetes in the face of high-level exercise. Each athlete is unique and will require individualized adjustments until an optimal routine is established.

In the setting of scholastic athletics, children may be prone to greater variability in blood glucose levels, and adolescents demonstrate hormonal changes, which can contribute to greater difficulty in controlling blood glucose levels as well. In this special group of diabetic athletes, it is vital to ensure that parents, coaches, teachers, and other adults understand the importance of scheduled meals, snacks, and adequate fluids, as well as appreciating the features and management of hypoglycemia.[42,43]

Blood Glucose Control

Type 1 diabetes

In general, T1D athletes exhibiting poor metabolic control (HgA_{1c} >9%) should refrain from moderate- or higher-level exercise until adequate blood sugar control has been obtained. This is prudent to avoid the risk of exacerbating hyperglycemia and to minimize the risk of progression to frank diabetic ketoacidosis (DKA).[44] The duration and intensity of exercise will determine the specific modifications that need to be made in the treatment regimen.

Adjustments in both dietary intake and insulin dosing are essential for optimal performance and prevention of deleterious glucose fluctuations. Waiting 60 to 90 minutes after a meal before exercising and monitoring blood glucose both during and after exercise/sport are important baseline management measures. With respect to diet, CHO-rich, low-glycemic-index (see later section) meals should be consumed 1 to 3 hours before exercise.[38,45] Immediately before and during an exercise bout, consumption of additional CHO (17 g at initiation and 17 g every 15 minutes for 60 minutes for exercise at 65% Vo_2 max) is beneficial in maintaining glucose levels during exercise and particularly after exercise in patients with both T1D and T2D.[46]

The consumption of a low-glycemic-index diet improves metabolic regulation,[47] because these foods require less insulin for optimal glucose utilization. Such foods give a low and slow glucose rise when consumed and include raw cornstarch, non-starchy vegetables, fruits, nuts, milk, and fructose and lactose sugars. Characteristic high-glycemic-index foods that give rise to rapid and high-glucose responses include white bread and glucose sugars.[48] Provided that the diet contains enough CHO (at least 35% of total calories) to maintain normal glycogen levels, low-calorie diets can be used in this population without affecting exercise tolerance.[49]

Comfort with insulin adjustments with exercise is essential for athletic success and prevention of acute complications. If pre-exercise blood glucose is 100 to 250 mg/dL, it is generally safe to begin exercising.[50] American Diabetes Association guidelines[42] for regulating the glycemic response to exercise include the following:

1. Metabolic control before exercise—avoid exercise if fasting glucose is greater than 250 mg/dL and ketosis is present; use caution if glucose is greater than 300 mg/dL with no ketosis; ingest added CHO if glucose levels are less than 100 mg/dL.
2. Blood glucose monitoring before and after exercise—identify when changes in insulin or food intake are necessary, and learn the glycemic response to different exercise conditions.
3. Food intake—consume added CHO to avoid hypoglycemia with exercise; CHO-rich foods should be readily available during and after exercise.

T1D athletes should avoid exercise during peak insulin times, and the dose of short- or rapid-acting insulin should be decreased by 30% to 50% if given before exercise.[42] Near euglycemia has been shown to be obtainable in T1D athletes during exercise even with reductions of 70% to 90% in insulin dose.[51] In fact, doses of insulin may also need to be further reduced 10% to 30% as an athlete becomes more fit.[52] For a morning workout, the dose of the athlete's short-acting insulin (regular insulin, onset 1–2 hours, peak 2–4 hours) should be reduced. For an afternoon workout or competition, the dose of the intermediate-acting insulin should be reduced (NPH insulin, onset 1–3 hours, peak 4–10 hours). Long-acting, peakless insulin such as insulin glargine should have the total dose reduced as above. Insulin absorption is more rapid and less predictable when injected into the leg before exercise.[53] The abdomen is the preferred site for athletes because of its ease of access during meals and more predictable absorption time.[54]

Special note should be made of high-intensity exercise as would be common with competitive sports. Such activity may elevate blood sugar levels in diabetics, but this response is generally temporary and results from a number of hormonal factors. Blood glucose levels usually fall for several hours after exercise, so such a transient increase after high-intensity workouts should not be treated with insulin.[55]

Insulin pumps

Athletes using insulin pumps should precede intense exercise by reducing the action of the pump by 50% about 1 hour before activity.[56] For lower-intensity activity, the standard basal rate may be maintained with a small reduction in the premeal bolus. If the insulin pump must be removed before contact/collision sport, it should be removed 30 minutes prior to exercise to compensate for the persistent insulin effect after pump removal. For prolonged activity more than 1 hour, small boluses may be needed to prevent a hypoinsulinemic state. Boluses should be given every hour, and the amount of insulin given should represent about 50% of the usual hourly basal rate.[33]

Type 2 diabetes

For T2D athletes, the primary goals for management include not only preserved performance and prevention of hypo- and hyperglycemia but also improved insulin sensitivity and uptake of glucose in skeletal muscle, with a concomitant improvement in postprandial blood glucose. The major metabolic problem for active T2D patients is a reduced capacity to store excess glucose as muscle glycogen.[57] Consequently, the most important effect of exercise for improving glucose regulation is the lowered glycogen storage in skeletal muscles.[45] Ideally, if energy stores remain low, the calories consumed in the next meal can be stored as glycogen rather than contributing to hyperglycemia.

T2D athletes on diet therapy alone should be able to exercise with no further caution than individuals with normal glucose tolerance provided no major vascular complications are present.[58] No pre-exercise CHO intake is necessary. In general, far lower CHO intake during exercise is required of T2D athletes, as these patients have a lower rate of glucose metabolism and a much lower risk of hypoglycemia with exercise training relative to T1D patients. CHO intake for these athletes should only be undertaken during exercise to prevent hypoglycemia, particularly as weight reduction is desirable, and limited CHO intake will be beneficial to this goal. The major adjustment for T2D athletes involves adjustment of oral hypoglycemic therapy as dictated by their glucose values. These medications are reviewed later in this article.

Postexercise

After exercise, glycogen resynthesis and storage occur in skeletal muscles and require insulin to be most efficient. This process is essential to allow the athlete to physically prepare for the next bout of high-level exertion. Repletion is faster after ingestion of high-glycemic-index foods such as glucose and sucrose rather than fructose.[59] After training, T1D athletes should immediately consume a high-CHO, high-glycemic-index meal with insulin to refill glycogen stores. Postexercise consumption should consist of 30 to 40 g of CHO for every 30 minutes of intense exercise[44] as part of the 500 to 600 g of CHO required daily in typical endurance athletes.[60] If adequate caloric intake does not occur, hypoglycemia may arise after exercise because of the increased insulin sensitivity of exercising skeletal muscles.[38,45] Restoration of glycogen stores normalizes insulin sensitivity. For extensive and/or late afternoon/evening exercise, blood glucose levels should be monitored once or twice during the night.

Children

Current ADA recommendations[50] for the management of T1D in active children include the following:

1. Eat 15 to 30 minutes before vigorous activity or activity of longer than 30 minutes duration (15 g of CHO are generally adequate for 30 minutes of moderate-intensity activity).
2. Always carry a CHO source.
3. Decrease insulin typically by 10% to 20% before sport activity, with adjustments over time based on glucose values and intensity of training.

Medications

Medication management of the diabetic athlete requires a delicate balance between maintenance of adequate glucose levels to allow for sport activity while minimizing the likelihood of hypoglycemia. Insulin and medications that stimulate insulin production increase the risk for hypoglycemia and must be used with caution in this population. The following subsection is a brief review of available medications for use in active diabetics.

Insulin

Insulin may be used by both T1D and T2D athletes. Insulin enhances the peripheral uptake of glucose primarily by muscle and liver while inhibiting glucose production and glycogenolysis. Insulin is available in short-acting forms (regular insulin, insulin lispro) for use at the time of caloric consumption as well as medium (NPH) and long-acting (insulin glargine) forms, which provide baseline glucose-controlling effect throughout the day. Because of its glucose-lowering effect, insulin dosing requires adjustment prior to exercise as addressed here.

In T2D patients, relative insulin deficiency is due to cellular resistance to insulin action at the levels of the muscle cell, the adipocyte, the hepatocyte, and the β cell [61] in addition to abnormally elevated glucagon. Medications for T2D thus target 3 major mechanisms: (1) impaired peripheral glucose uptake (liver, fat, muscle), (2) excessive hepatic glucose release (with elevated glucagon), and (3) insufficient insulin secretion.[62]

Insulin sensitizers

Biguanides (metformin) and thiazolidinediones (TZD) (rosiglitazone, pioglitazone) specifically target insulin resistance. Metformin enhances the sensitivity of both peripheral (primarily muscle) and hepatic tissues to insulin. It also inhibits hepatic gluconeogenesis and glycogenolysis. TZDs improve insulin sensitization at the level of muscle and adipocyte by activating peroxisome proliferators-activated gamma receptors (PPAR-gamma).[62] Because of their mechanism of action, these agents do not place patients at risk for hypoglycemia and can be safely used without dosage adjustment before or after exercise.

Insulin secretagogues

These agents primarily address the progressive decline in β-cell function seen in T2D diabetes. Sulfonylurea agents (glipizide, glyburide, glimepiride, chlorpropamide) are best used as an adjunct to insulin sensitizer therapy to achieve goal levels of control. Sulfonylureas enhance insulin secretion after binding to specific receptors on β cells. Receptor activation leads to closure of a potassium-dependent ATP channel, leading to decreased potassium influx and depolarization of the β-cell membrane. Sulfonylureas suppress hepatic glucose production as well.[63]

Glinides are newer insulin secretagogues, which include repaglinide, a meglitinide, and the amino acid derivative nateglinide. Each is taken before meals and acts rapidly to increase insulin production in an effort to restore premeal glucose levels and control postprandial glucose. They do not need to be taken if meals are missed, or dosing can be skipped if exercise follows the meal.

In general, insulin secretagogues should be half-dosed on days of exercise, particularly if the athlete is near "goal HgA$_{1c}$", as their hypoglycemic risk will be correspondingly higher. Nonetheless, the severity of hypoglycemia with these agents is, in general, low.

Carbohydrate-absorption blockers (alpha-glucosidase [α-glucosidase] inhibitors)

Acarbose and miglitol are taken before meals to reduce glucose absorption, decrease meal-associated blood glucose elevations, and thus reduce the required insulin response. The usefulness of this class of medications can be limited by gastrointestinal discomfort and variability in gastric emptying. They can be useful in addition to combination oral therapy or in patients with mild fasting hyperglycemia.

Incretin potentiators

Glucagon-like peptide-1 gut-derived incretin hormone stimulates insulin, suppresses hepatic glucose release, inhibits gastric emptying, and reduces appetite and food intake. Exenatide is injected subcutaneously twice daily, is approved for use in combination with sulfonylureas, metformin, or both,[62] and is not associated with weight gain. Exenatide does not appear to increase the risk of hypoglycemia unless used in combination with a sulfonylurea. It also does not blunt the glucagon response to hypoglycemia, and no dose adjustment is warranted before exercise.

Dipeptidyl peptidase IV (DDP-4) inhibitors target both excess glucagon and inadequate postmeal insulin secretion. Sitagliptin was the first approved DDP-4 inhibitor, having shown the ability to enhance normal insulin action while suppressing glucagon during a meal. The overall incidence of hypoglycemia with DDP-4 inhibitors is equal to that with placebo,[62] and there is no dose adjustment necessary before, during, or after exercise.

On-Field Management of Complications

Hypoglycemia

Hypoglycemia may arise for many reasons in the active population. Common causes include too high a daily dose of insulin or oral hypoglycemics, errors in dosage, increased activity duration or intensity, insufficient or delayed food intake, and alcohol intake during or immediately after exercise. As glycogen is used during exercise, the reduced glycogen concentration increases insulin action. Although the rate of CHO utilization depends on the intensity and duration of exercise, training status, and prior diet, as glycogen stores in active muscles and liver are depleted, the risk for hypoglycemia correspondingly increases.[64]

Diabetic athletes with prior episodes of hypoglycemia generally demonstrate blunted neuroendocrine (glucagon, insulin, catecholamines) and metabolic (endogenous glucose production, lipolysis, ketogenesis) counter-regulatory responses during subsequent exercise.[65,66] This "counter-regulatory failure mechanism" is postulated to be the result of cortisol stimulation that occurs during a stress such as hypoglycemia and the effect that it exerts on the central nervous system.[10] These individuals maintain a higher susceptibility to hypoglycemia in the future.

Pre-exercise prevention

In T1D athletes, adjustments in insulin dosing are needed prior to exercise, but adequate CHO replacement during and after exercise appears to have the most profound effect on preventing hypoglycemia.[67] If the insulin schedule is not altered before exercise, a CHO snack must be ingested to minimize the likelihood of hypoglycemia.[68]

Individualization of insulin dosing, timing, and caloric intake before, during, and after exercise is critical. Decreasing 1 U of regular insulin from the usual dose or adding 15 g of CHO increases blood glucose by approximately 50 mg/dL.[69] As noted earlier, hypoglycemia during exercise can be minimized by reducing the typical insulin dose by 30% to 50%. If exercise is beyond 60 minutes, insulin dose must be reduced by 80% of the initial dose in T1D athletes.[70] Decreased insulin dose is not always possible to anticipate, because exercise is often unplanned, particularly in children. Diet modification takes on additional significance in this group.

As stated above, no major dietary adjustments are necessary for T2D athletes. Those using oral hypoglycemics may need to adjust their dosing based on the relative risk of hypoglycemia inherent in the therapy that they are taking.

Management of acute hypoglycemia

Patients and providers should readily recognize the symptoms of hypoglycemia (glucose <70 mg/dL): dizziness, weakness, sweating, headache, hunger, pallor, blurred vision, slurred speech, confusion, irritability, and poor coordination. If hypoglycemia occurs, exercise should be stopped, and blood sugar should be monitored every 15 minutes until it rises above 80 mg/dL. Acute hypoglycemia should be treated immediately with 15 g of CHO: 1/2 cup of fruit juice, 4 glucose tablets, 6 oz of sweetened carbonated beverage, or 8 oz of low-fat milk.[71] Special note should be made that patients using α-glucosidase inhibitors (acarbose or miglitol) concurrently with insulin or insulin secretagogues will require treatment with glucose, because these agents prevent rapid absorption of nonglucose CHO.[50]

More pronounced hypoglycemia may require intravenous glucose, and severe hypoglycemia should be treated with glucagon 1 mg subcutaneously or intramuscularly to produce a rapid release of liver glycogen. It should be noted that this therapy is ineffective if all liver glycogen stores have been depleted by prolonged, intense exercise.

Late-onset postexercise hypoglycemia

The risk of hypoglycemia in insulin-treated patients persists long after strenuous exercise via several mechanisms. Late-onset postexercise hypoglycemia (LOPEH) has been seen in T1D 6 to 24 hours after activity.[72] After exertion, muscle and hepatic glycogen stores are filled by using circulating plasma glucose. That, coupled with increased insulin sensitivity and glucose uptake by peripheral tissues and a blunting of the glucoregulatory response to insulin-induced hypoglycemia, may lead to late-onset hypoglycemia, often nocturnal.[44] This syndrome most commonly occurs with increases in training level or during 2-a-day practices during preseason, although it may occur at any time.

Research in this area demonstrated that regardless of postexercise supplementation, glucose concentrations fell after 22.00 hours, and prebedtime snacks were important for helping to correct or avoid nocturnal hypoglycemia.[68] Consumption of any commercially available sports drink has been shown to be effective in helping to avoid LOPEH; however, sports drinks with a mix of CHO, fat, and protein were associated with sustained hyperglycemia (and lack of hypoglycemia) during most of the postexercise period.[68] This late-onset hypoglycemia is also effectively prevented by whole milk[68] and slowly absorbed snacks, such as chips, chocolate, and most fruits.

Hyperglycemia

Frank hyperglycemia in athletes (>250 mg/dL) occurs more commonly in T1D generally as a result of low circulating insulin levels. Hyperglycemia may also result from inadequate insulin administration, excessive food intake, inactivity, failure to take oral hypoglycemics, illness, stress, or injury.

If pre-exercise blood glucose is more than 250 mg/dL, T1D athletes should check for urinary ketones. If ketonuria is moderate to high, exercise should be avoided until glucose values improve and ketones resolve. Aggressive lowering of blood glucose in these patients may prevent development of ketoacidosis. It has been suggested that T1D athletes with moderate hyperglycemia (250–300 mg/dL) but no ketones may exercise as long as they monitor their glucose every 15 minutes and demonstrate that glucose values are falling.[50]

Patients with T2D should avoid exercise if blood glucose values are more than 400 mg/dL. The key differentiation between T1D and T2D diabetics with exercise is the risk of ketosis and acidosis in T1D patients with relatively inadequate insulin and poorly controlled blood glucose. Individuals with T2D demonstrate hyperglycemia primarily from overeating or poor glucose utilization from insulin resistance and/or insufficient activity.

SUMMARY

Although regular exercise is a pivotal component of management in diabetics, the demands of sports and competition can predispose athletes with diabetes to potentially harmful complications such as hypo- and hyperglycemia. A basic understanding of substrate metabolism, special nutritional needs, blood glucose control, medications, and management of on-field complications in athletes with diabetes is important for medical professionals charged with the daily care of diabetic athletes. Individual metabolic responses to exercise, differences in diets and timing of meals, the interplay between various stressors of daily life, anxiety provoked by the anticipation of competition, and varying medications and doses preclude the development of a "generalized" algorithm for the daily management of diabetic athletes. "Individualized" management strategies should be developed only after consultation with a team of medical professionals, including the athletic trainer, sports nutritionist, and physician.

REFERENCES

1. Albright A, Franz M, Hornsby G, et al. American College of Sports Medicine position stand. Exercise and type 2 diabetes. Med Sci Sports Exerc 2000;32(7): 1345–60.
2. Association AD. Physical activity/exercise and diabetes. Diabetes Care 2004; 27(Supplement 1):S58–62.
3. Sigal RJ, Kenny GP, Wasserman DH, et al. Physical activity/exercise and type 2 diabetes - A consensus statement from the American diabetes association. Diabetes Care 2006;29(6):1433–8.
4. King H, Aubert RE, Herman WH. Global burden of diabetes, 1995–2025-Prevalence, numerical estimates, and projections. Diabetes Care 1998;21(9):1414–31.
5. Deckelbaum RJ, Williams CL. Childhood obesity: the health issue. Obesity 2001; 9:s239–43.
6. Unger J. Management of type 1 diabetes. Prim Care 2007;34(4):791–808.
7. Chamberlain J. Type 2 Diabetes - 30 years of progress. Available at: www. nih.goc/about/researchresultsforthepublic/type2Diabetes.pdf.
8. DeFronzo RA. Pathogenesis of type 2 diabetes mellitus. Med Clin North Am 2004; 88(4):787–835.
9. Marliss EB, Vranic M. Intense exercise has unique, effects on both insulin release and its roles in glucoregulation. Implications for diabetes. Diabetes 2002; 51(Suppl1):S271–83.
10. Camacho RC, Galassetti P, Davis SN, et al. Glucoregulation during and after exercise in health and insulin-dependent diabetes. Exerc Sport Sci Rev 2005;33(1): 17–23 OD - 2005/01/11.
11. Rockl KS, Witczak CA, Goodyear LJ. Signaling mechanisms in skeletal muscle: acute responses and chronic adaptations to exercise. IUBMB Life 2008;60(3): 145–53 OD - 2008/04/02.

12. Rattigan S, Wheatley C, Richards SM, et al. Exercise and insulin-mediated capillary recruitment in muscle. Exerc Sport Sci Rev 2005;33(1):43–8 OD - 2005/01/11.
13. Richter EA, Ploug T, Galbo H. Increased muscle glucose uptake after exercise. No need for insulin during exercise. Diabetes 1985;34(10):1041–8 OD - 1985/10/01.
14. Constable SH, Favier RJ, Cartee GD, et al. Muscle glucose transport: interactions of in vitro contractions, insulin, and exercise. J Appl Physiol 1988;64(6):2329–32 OD - 1988/06/01.
15. Ivy JL. The insulin-like effect of muscle contraction. Exerc Sport Sci Rev 1987;15: 29–51 OD - 1987/01/01.
16. Lehmann R, Kaplan V, Bingisser R, et al. Impact of physical activity on cardiovascular risk factors in IDDM. Diabetes Care 1997;20(10):1603–11 OD - 1997/10/07.
17. Riddell M, Perkins B. Type 1 diabetes and exercise part I: applications of exercise physiology to patient management during vigorous activity. Can J Diabetes 2006; 30:63–71.
18. Fuchsjager-Mayrl G, Pleiner J, Wiesinger GF, et al. Exercise training improves vascular endothelial function in patients with type 1 diabetes. Diabetes Care 2002;25(10):1795–801 OD - 2002/09/28.
19. Church TS, LaMonte MJ, Barlow CE, et al. Cardiorespiratory fitness and body mass index as predictors of cardiovascular disease mortality among men with diabetes. Arch Intern Med 2005;165(18):2114–20 OD - 2005/10/12.
20. Chamoon H, Duffy H, Fleischer N, et al. The effect of intensive treatment of diabetes on the development and progression of long-term complications in insulin-dependent diabetes mellitus. N Engl J Med 1993;329:977–86.
21. Jimenez CC, Corcoran MH, Crawley JT, et al. National athletic trainers' association position statement: management of the athlete with type 1 diabetes mellitus. J Athl Train 2007;42(4):536–45 OD - 2008/04/25.
22. Knowler WC, Barrett-Connor E, Fowler SE, et al. Reduction in the incidence of type 2 diabetes with lifestyle intervention or metformin. N Engl J Med 2002; 346(6):393–403 OD - 2002/02/08.
23. Franz M. Nutrition, physical activity, and diabetes. In: Ruderman N, Devlin JT, Schneider SH, editors. Handbook of exercise in diabetes. Alexandria (VA): American Diabetes Association, Inc.; 2002. p. 321–37.
24. Joint Position Statement of the American College of Sports Medicine, The American Dietetic Association and Dietitians of Canada: nutrition and athletic performance. J Am Diet Assoc 2000;12:1543–56.
25. Neufer PD, Costill DL, Flynn MG, et al. Improvements in exercise performance effects of carbohydrate feeding and diet. J Appl Physiol 1987;62:983–8.
26. Wright D, Sherman W, Dernbach A. Carbohydrate feedings before, during, or in combination improve cycling endurance performance. J Appl Physiol 1991;71: 1082–8.
27. Sherman WM, Costill DL, Fink WJ, et al. The effect of exercise and diet manipulation on muscle glycogen and its subsequent use during performance. Int J Sports Med 1981;2:114–8.
28. Nathan D, Madnek S, Delahanty L. Programming pre-exercise snacks to prevent post-exercise hypoglycemia in intensively treated insulin-dependent diabetics. Ann Intern Med 1985;4:483–6.
29. Coggan A, Swanson S. Nutritional manipulation before and during exercise effects on performance. Med Sci Sports Exerc 1992;24:S331–5.
30. Sherman WM, Doyle JA, Lamb DR, et al. Dietary carbohydrate, muscle glycogen, and exercise performance during 7 d of training. Am J Clin Nutr 1993;57:27–31.

31. Coyle E, Montain S. Benefits of fluid replacement with carbohydrate during exercise. Med Sci Sports Exerc 1992;24:S324–30.
32. Ivy JL, Katz AL, Cutler CL, et al. Muscle glycogen synthesis after exercise: effect of time of carbohydrate ingestion. J Appl Physiol 1988;64:480–5.
33. Schiffrin A, Parikh S. Accommodating planned exercise in type 1 diabetes patients on intensive treatment. Diabetes Care 1985;8:337–42.
34. Gonder-Frederick L. Hypoglycemia. In: Franz MJ, editor. A core curriculum for diabetes education: diabetes management therapies. Chicago: American Association of Diabetes Educators; 2001. p. 279–306.
35. United States Department of Health and Human Services. Dietary Guidelines for Americans. 2005.
36. Eisenstein J, Roberts SB, Dallal G, et al. High protein weight-loss diets: are they safe and do they work? A review of experimental and epidemiologic data. Nutr Rev 2002;60:189–200.
37. Kenefick RW, Hazzard MP, Mahood NV, et al. Thirst sensations and AVP responses at rest and during exercise-cold exposure. Med Sci Sports Exerc 2004;36(9):1528–34.
38. Horton E. Role and management of exercise in diabetes mellitus. Diabetes Care 1988;11:201–11.
39. Ebeling P, Tuominen JA, Bourey R, et al. Athletes with IDDM exhibit impaired metabolic control and increased lipid utilization with no increase in insulin sensitivity. Diabetes 1995;44:471–7.
40. Cuff DJ, Meneilly GS, Martin A, et al. Effective exercise modality to reduce insulin resistance in women with type 2 diabetes. Diabetes Care 2003;26:2977–82.
41. Maiorana A, O'Driscoll G, Goodman C, et al. Combined aerobic and resistance exercise improves glycemic control and fitness in type 2 diabetes. Diabetes Res Clin Pract 2002;56:115–23.
42. Association AD. Diabetes mellitus and exercise. [position statement]. Diabetes Care 2002;25(Suppl 1):S64.
43. Association AD. Care of children with diabetes in the school and day care setting. [position statement]. Diabetes Care 2002;25(Suppl 1):S122–5.
44. Lisle DK, Trojian TH. Managing the athlete with type 1 diabetes. Current Sports Med Rep 2006;5:93–8.
45. Jensen J, Leighton B. The diabetic athlete. In: M. RJ, editor. Nutrition in sport. Oxford (UK): Blackwell Science; 2000. p. 457–66.
46. Tamis-Jortberg B, Downs D, Colten M. Effects of a glucose polymer sports drink on blood glucose, insulin, and performance in subjects with diabetes. Diabetes Educ 1996;22:471–8.
47. Ludwig D. The glycemic index: physiological mechanisms relating to obesity, diabetes, and cardiovascular disease. JAMA 2002;287:2414–23.
48. Foster-Powell K, Miller JB. International tables of glycemic index. Am J Clin Nutr 1995;62:871S–90S.
49. Bogardus C, LaGrange B, Horton E, et al. Comparison of carbohydrate-containing and carbohydrate-restricted hypocaloric diets in the treatment of obesity: endurance and metabolic fuel homeostasis during strenuous exercise. J Clin Invest 1981;68:399–404.
50. Flood L, Constance A. Diabetes & exercise safety. Am J Nurs 2002;102(6):47–55.
51. Mauvais-Jarvis F, Sobngwi E, Porcher R, et al. Glucose response to intense aerobic exercise in type 1 diabetes: maintenance of near euglycemia despite a drastic decrease in insulin dose. Diabetes Care 2003;26:1316–7.

52. Devlin J, Ruderman N, editors. The health professionals guide to diabetes and exercise. Alexandria (VA): American Diabetes Association; 1995.
53. Koivisto VA, Felig P. Effects of leg exercise on insulin absorption in diabetic patients. N Engl J Med 1978;298:77–83.
54. Frid A, Ostman J, Linde B. Hypoglycemia risk during exercise after intramuscular injection of insulin in the thigh of IDDM. Diabetes Care 1990;8:337–43.
55. Franz M, editor. A core curriculum for diabetes education. 4th edition. Chicago: American Association of Diabetes Educators; 2001. p. 22.
56. Sonnenberg GE, Kemmer FW, Berger M. Exercise in type I diabetic patients treated with continuous subcutaneous insulin infusion. Prevention of exercise induced hypoglycemia. Diabetologia 1990;33:696–703.
57. Shulman GI, Rothman D, Jue T, et al. Quantification of muscle glycogen synthesis in normal subjects and subjects with non-insulin-dependent diabetes by 13C nuclear magnetic resonance spectroscopy. N Engl J Med 1990;322:223–8.
58. Zinker B. Nutrition and exercise in individuals with diabetes. Clin Sports Med 1999;18(3):585–606.
59. Blom PCS, Hostmark AT, Vaage O, et al. Effect of different post-exercise sugar diets on the rate of muscle glycogen synthesis. Med Sci Sports Exerc 1987;19: 491–6.
60. Ivy J. Muscle glycogen synthesis before and after exercise. Sports Med 1991;11: 6–19.
61. Kahn SE, Porte D Jr. Pathophysiology of type 2 diabetes mellitus. In: SR, Porte D Jr, editors. Diabetes mellitus. Stamfort (CT): Appleton and Lange; 1997. p. 487–512.
62. McDonnell M. Combination therapy with new targets in type 2 diabetes. J Cardiopulm Rehabil Prev 2007;27:193–201.
63. Groop L, Luzi L, Melander A, et al. Different effects of glibenclamide and glipizide on insulin secretion and hepatic glucose production in normal and NIDDM subjects. Diabetes 1987;36:1320–8.
64. Coyle E. Substrate utilization during exercise in active people. Am J Clin Nutr 1995;61:968S–79S.
65. Cryer PE, Davis S, Shamoon H. Hypoglycemia in diabetes. Diabetes Care 2003; 26:1902–12.
66. Galassetti P, Tate D, Neill RA, et al. Effect of antecedent hypoglycemia on counterregulatory responses to subsequent euglycemic exercise in type 1 diabetes. Diabetes 2003;52:1761–9.
67. Grimm JJ, Ybarra J, Berne C, et al. A new table for prevention of hypoglycemia during physical activity in type 1 diabetic patients. Diabetes Metab 2004;30: 465–70.
68. Hernandez JM, Moccia T, Fluckey JD, et al. Fluid snacks to help persons with type I diabetes avoid late onset postexercise hypoglycemia. Med Sci Sports Exerc 2000;32:904–10.
69. Boswell E, Davis D, Partin L, et al. The activity activity: a tool for teaching how to adjust for exercise variations. Diabetes Educ 1997;23:63–6.
70. Kemmer F, Berger M. Therapy and better quality of life: the dichotomous role of exercise in diabetes mellitus. Diabetes Metab Rev 1986;2:53–68.
71. Funnell M, editor. A core curriculum for diabetes education. 3rd edition. Chicago: American Association of Diabetes Educators; 1998. p. 32.
72. Peirce N. Diabetes and exercise. Br J Sports Med 1999;33:161–73.

Index

Note: Page numbers of article titles are in **boldface** type.

Clin Sports Med 28 (2009) 497–504
doi:10.1016/S0278-5919(09)00034-9
0278-5919/09/$ – see front matter © 2009 Elsevier Inc. All rights reserved.

sportsmed.theclinics.com

Moving?

Make sure your subscription moves with you!

To notify us of your new address, find your **Clinics Account Number** (located on your mailing label above your name), and contact customer service at:

E-mail: elspcs@elsevier.com

800-654-2452 (subscribers in the U.S. & Canada)
314-453-7041 (subscribers outside of the U.S. & Canada)

Fax number: 314-523-5170

Elsevier Periodicals Customer Service
11830 Westline Industrial Drive
St. Louis, MO 63146

*To ensure uninterrupted delivery of your subscription, please notify us at least 4 weeks in advance of move.

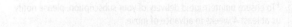

Printed and bound by CPI Group (UK) Ltd, Croydon, CR0 4YY

03/10/2024

01040464-0012